Exercise and Fitness – Benefits and Risks

Exercise and Fitness-Benefits and Risks

Children & Exercise XVIII

Edited by

Karsten Froberg
Ole Lammert
Henrik St. Hansen
Cameron J.R. Blimkie

Odense University Press 1997

Exercise and Fitness – Benefits and Risks is published with the
generous support of The Danish Ministry of Culture

© The authors and Odense University Press 1997
Printed by Special-Trykkeriet Viborg, Denmark
Cover design by Maja Honoré
ISBN 87-7838-322-6

All photos in this book – including the cover illustrations – by
Niels Nyholm, who has copyright to the material.

Odense University Press
Campusvej 55
DK-5230 Odense M

Phone +45 66 15 79 99
Fax +45 66 15 81 26
E-mail: press@forlag.ou.dk
Internet-location: http://www.ou.dk/press

RJ
133
E9Y
1997

Contents

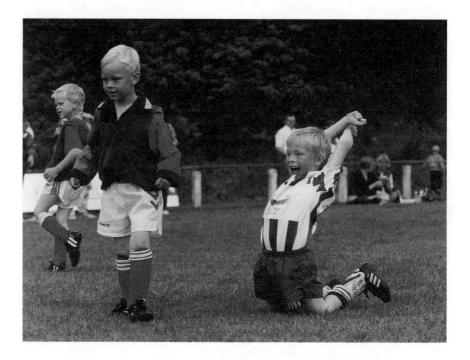

Contributors

Oded Bar-Or
Children's Exercise and Nutrition
Centre
Chedoke Hospital Division
McMaster University
Hamilton – Ontario L8N 3Z5
Canada

Per-Olof Åstrand
Karolinska Institutet
Institut för Fysiology III
Box 5626
S-114 86 Stockholm
Sweden

Thorkild I. A. Sørensen
Institut for Sygdomsforebyggelse
Kommunehospitalet
Østre Farimagsgade 5
1399 København K
Denmark

James N. Roemmich, Pamela A. Clark
and Alan D. Rogol
Health Science Center, Department of
Pediatric
University of Virginia
Box 386
Charlottesville VA 22908
U.S.A.

Jorunn Sundgot-Borgen and R. Bahr
Norwegian University of Sport and
Physical Education
Box 4014 Ulleval Hageby,
0806 Oslo, Norway

Alex F. Roche
Division of Human Biology
Wright State University
1005 Xenia Avenue
Yellow Springs, Ohio 45387-1695
U.S.A.

Henrik Steen Hansen
Medical Department B
Odense University Hospital
5000 Odense C
Denmark

Frank M. Galioto Jr.
Child Cardiology Associates
Georgetown University
3299 Woodburn Road, Suite 460
Annandale, VA 22003
U.S.A.

Cameron J.R. Blimkie and Suzi
Kriemler
Department of Kinesiology
McMaster University
Hamilton, Ontario, L8S 4K1
Canada

Han C. G. Kemper
EMGO Institute
Faculty of Medicine
Vrije Universiteit
Van der Boechorststraat 7
1081 BT Amsterdam
The Netherlands

Robert M. Malina
Michigan State University
Institute for the Study of Youth Sports
East Lansing, Michigan
U.S.A.

Neil Armstrong and Joanne Welsman
Children's Health and Exercise
Research Centre
University of Exeter
Exeter EXI 2LU
United Kingdom

Thomas W. Rowland
Baystate Medical Center
759 Chestnut Street
Springfield, Massachusetts 01199
U.S.A.

Gaston Beunen
Faculty of Physical Education and
Physiotherapy
Catholic University of Leuven
Tervuursevest 101
B-3001 Heverlee
Belgium

Willem van Mechelen
EMGO Institute
Faculty of Medicine
Vrije Universiteit
Van der Boechorststraat 7
1081 BT Amsterdam
The Netherlands

Yngvar Ommundsen
Norwegian University of Sport and
Physical Education
Box 4014 Ulleval Hageby,
0806 Oslo
Norway

Editors:
Karsten Froberg
Institute of Physical Education
Faculty of Health Sciences
Odense University
Campusvej 55
5230 Odense M
Denmark

Ole Lammert
Institute of Physical Education
Faculty of Health Sciences
Odense University
Campusvej 55
5230 Odense M
Denmark

Henrik Steen Hansen
Institute of Physical Education
Faculty of Health Sciences
Odense University
Campusvej 55
5230 Odense M
Denmark

Cameron (Joe) Blimkie
Children's Hospital, Institute of Sports
Medicine
Hainsworth Street, Westmead
NSW 2145
PO Box 3515 Parramatta
NSW 2124
Australia
(Present address)

Preface

Exercise and Fitness – Benefits and Risks, is a book of chapters by world authorities on selected topics with a common theme of children and exercise. All chapters were presented as invited lectures or at workshops at the XVIII symposium of the European Group of Pediatric Work Physiology, hosted by the Institute of Physical Education, Faculty of Health Sciences, Odense University at Interscan Hotel Faaborg Fjord, Denmark, in September 1995.

The European Group of Pediatric Work Physiology (EGPWP) is an informal organized yet highly commited group of pediatric clinicians and researchers in exercise physiology, physical education, biomechanics, and rehabilitative medicine. The EGPWP has hosted biennial scientific meetings and published conference proceedings since 1967. Most of the meetings has been held in Europe, with the exception of meetings in Israel in 1972, in Quebec in 1979, and in Toronto in 1993, where the first joint meeting of EGPWP and The North American Society of Pediatric Exercise Medicine (NASPEM) took place. EGPWP has always had very good relations and collaborations with researchers in the pediatric field from mostly North America, Australia and New Zealand, especially after the formel foundation in 1986 of NASPEM.

The purpose of the conference in Faaborg was as always in EGPWP meetings, to bring together scholars from the whole world, who have common interest in children, physical activity and health. Besides providing a presentation forum for young scientists and researchers, the conference also provided the opportunity for the exchange of international perspectives and interdisciplinary dialogue among leading researchers and practitioners in the relatively new subdiscipline of Pediatric Exercise Science.

The conference was also organised to celebrate the 25th anniversary of the Institute of Physical Education, Odense University, whose research interest for years have dealt with Exercise and Fitness – Benefits and Risks, with special reference to children.

The text is organized into 16 chapters. The introductory chapter by Oded Bar-Or is dedicated to the memory of Dr. Joseph Rutenfranz, one of the founding members of the EGPWP, for his contributions to the development of Pediatric Exercise Science in general and the EGPWP in particular. It discuss the increasing evidence that an enhanced physical activity can induce several physiological, psycho-social and medical benefits to the child with a chronic disease. Chapter two by Per-Olof

Åstrand addresses future research directions, ask questions – and give some answers in relation to: – risks for the children; – the importance of physical activity during those years for optimal development, for prevention of disease; – DNA technique, can it identify those, at high risks so that programmes can be individualised? – specific activities, can we find activities which can improve motor skills, and help children with problems in reading and writing? The third chapter by Thorkild I.A. Sørensen focus on the study of genes and environment, which provides better understanding of disease causation, better prediction of disease risks, and better assessment of environmental factors. James N. Roemmich, Pamela A. Clark and Alan D. Rogol, argue how sport training affect the normal physiology, growth and development, in childhood and adolescence, and if there is data which can define the influence of the hormonal mechanism. Jorunn Sundgot-Borgen and R. Bahr present data on subclinical and eating disorders in young athletes and discuss the risk factors and the aetiology in relation to athletes at different levels of sport participation and different sports. Alex F. Roche present data from the Fels Longitudinal Study about tracking in body composition and risk factors for cardiovascular disease from childhood to middle age. In the 7th chapter, Henrik St. Hansen overview the data on physical activity and blood pressure in children, and discuss the effectiveness and implications of physical activity as an important nonpharmacological approach to primary prevention of coronary heart disease. Frank M. Galioto Jr. goes through the etiologies of sudden death in the young. The etiologies can be divided into seven basic categories, which are presented with reference to incidence, treatment and prevention. Cameron J.R. Blimkie and Suzi Kriemler presents a number of relatively safe and highly precise techniques, which permit non-invasive evaluation of bone mineral status in children. The effect of puberty, the timing of peak bone density, fracture epidemiology, and the implications of developmental changes in bone mineralization and physical activity patterns on fracture risk during childhood and adolescence are discussed. In chapter ten Han C. G. Kemper focus on the effect of nutrition and physical activity on the growing skeleton. Robert M. Malina discuss the relationship between physical activity and physical fitness. The normal assumption is that the two are related and he try to answer the questions: Are the more active likely to be more fit? – Are the more fit likely to be more active? – And, is there a link between activity and fitness during childhood and youth and activity and fitness in adulthood? In the same area, Neil Armstrong and Joanne Welsman present an update on the assessment and interpretation of aerobic fitness in children and adolescents. In Thomas W. Rowlands chapter the focus is placed on aerobic trainability of athletic and non-athletic children, and he addresses the questions: How aerobically 'trainable' are prepubertal athletes? – Are there quantitative and qualitative difference in response to aerobic training between pre- and post-pubertal athletes? – How do such responses in maximal oxygen uptake translate into changes in endurance performance? In chapter fourteen Gaston Beunen considers the muscular strength development in children and adolescents. Age changes, sexual differences, variation within European populations and changes over time are discussed. In chapter fifteen, Willem van Mechelen gives an overview of the aetiology and prevention of sports injuries in youth – and finally the last chapter by Yngvar Ommundsen gives an overview of some of the literature on motivational aspects of sport for children and youth as well as some practical recommendations for sport practitioners derived from research reviewed.

Issues in Exercise and Fitness – Benefits and Risks is a compilation of state-of-the-art reviews by leading authorities on selected topics of relevance to clinicians, practitioners, and researchers who are interested in the effects of exercise in the growing child. It is not intended as, nor does it pretend to be, a comprehensive collection of all possible exercise issues. Nevertheless, this text adds significantly to the body of knowledge in this area and contributes to the further advancement of the still growing subdiscipline of Pediatric Exercise Science.

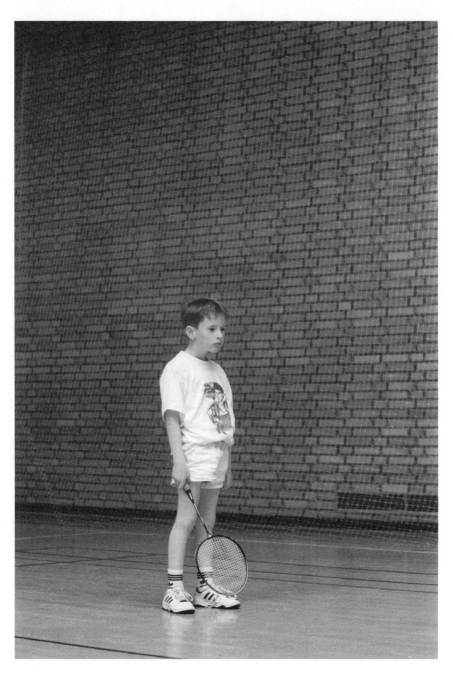

Acknowledgements

The editors thank the European Group of Pediatric Work Physiology and the North American Society of Pediatric Exercise Medicine for their great support.
The conference would not have been the success it was without the untiring help and great effort from the following members of the Conference Organisers :
Bjarne Andersen, Lars Elbæk, Jesper Franch, Lone Holm Petersen, Kaj Jensen, Addy Grue Jepsen, Klavs Madsen, Line Beese Rasmussen, Jørgen Povlsen, Lis Puggaard, Brit Thobo-Carlsen and Elisabeth Vang. Thanks also to special consultant Jonna Rose Rasmussen, Interscan Hotel Faaborg Fjord, for her expertise in planning and implementing the conference.
The editors would also like to thank all the chairpersons of both the free communications and symposia for their assistance and support.
Finally the editors would like to provide recognition and extend their appreciation to the following conference supporters. The success of the conference was largely dependent on the combined support from these sponsors and exhibitors.

Sponsors

The Danish Health Science Research Foundation
The Danish Ministry of Culture
Faculty of Health Sciences, Odense University
Team Danmark
The Municipality of Odense
Scandinavian Airlines System, SAS
The Danish Heart Foundation
The Danish Sports Research Council
Danish Association of Sports Medicine

Exhibitors

Innovision A/S
Power Sport

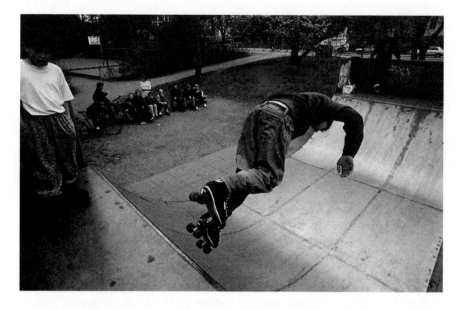

Chapter 1

Safe Exercise for the Child With a Chronic Disease

Oded Bar-Or

Introduction

It is with deep gratitude that I have accepted the invitation to present the Joseph Rutenfranz Lecture at the 1995 meeting of the Pediatric Work Physiology group (PWP). Indeed, it is an honour to be considered a suitable speaker for this prestigeous lectureship.

Prof. Dr. Joseph Rutenfranz, in addition to being one of the founders and pillars of PWP, has contributed widely as a scientist and author to various areas within pediatric exercise physiology and pediatric exercise medicine. During the last years of his life, Joseph devoted considerable attention to the potentially detrimental effects of sports participation among children and to the ethical implications therein. It is this aspect of his interest that I kept in mind when choosing the topic for this presentation.

Recent years have seen an increase in attention to the relevance of physical activity (PA) and of a sedentary lifestyle to the child with a chronic disease. As a result, exercise prescription has become an accepted therapeutic modality in several pediatric diseases and illnesses. Indeed, enhanced PA can induce specific and nonspecific benefits to the physical and mental health and well-being of children and adolescents with conditions such as asthma (Orenstein, 1996), cystic fibrosis (Cerny & Armitage, 1989), obesity (Bar-Or & Baranowski, 1994), diabetes mellitus (Dorchy & Poortmans, 1996), status post-surgery for congenital heart defects (Barber, 1995; Perrault, 1995), hypertension (Dlin, 1996) and neuromuscular disabilities (Steadward & Wheeler, 1996).

Yet, similar to other therapies, enhanced PA may entail risk to the child's health. Recognition of such risk and the means of preventing or ameliorating it is of paramount importance. The motto *CAUSE NO HARM* is as valid for exercise therapy as it is for any other therapy.

This presentation will start by a brief overview of apparent and real deleterious effects of exercise to the child with a chronic disease. This will be followed by a closer analysis of the means by which deleterious effects of enhanced PA can be prevented in three of the more common pediatric chronic diseases: Asthma, cystic fibrosis (CF) and insulin-dependent diabetes mellitus (IDDM). For an in-depth analysis of the interactions between exercise and these three diseases the reader can consult comprehensive reviews by Orenstein (1996), Cerny & Armitage

(1989) and Dorchy & Poortmans (1996). The current presentation will focus on work done in the author's laboratories at the Wingate Institute, Israel and the Children's Exercise & Nutrition Centre, Canada, in the context of contribution by other groups.

Deleterious effects of exercise: An overview

Table 1 is a summary of deleterious effects of exercise that have been documented or suggested in children with a chronic disease. While beneficial effects are usually induced by a chronic program of enhanced PA (often referred to as training or conditioning), and only seldom by an acute bout of exercise (e.g., enhanced mucus clearance in cystic fibrosis), it is the latter that induces most of the deleterious effects. Some effects, such as ischemic changes in the myocardium of a child with aortic stenosis, or oxygen desaturation in cystic fibrosis, result from unmet increased physiological demands during exercise (increased myocardial metabolic level and increased need for oxygen diffusion in the lungs, in the above two examples, respectively). As such, they usually occur when the activity is intense. Other abnormal changes, such as an epileptic seizure, exercise-induced asthma, or an anaphylactic response to exercise, are most probably mediated through triggers other than an high physiologic strain and they may occur with activities that are not necessarily intense.

Table 1: Deleterious effects of exertion in the child with a chronic disease	
Manifestation	**Underlying Condition**
Bronchoconstriction	Asthma, Atopy, C.F., Obesity
Chest Pain	Chest wall origin, Asthma, Mitral Valve Prolapse, Aortic Stenosis Kawasaki
Cramps	McArdle, Muscular Dystrophy, Myoglobinuria
Dehydration	C.F., Diabetes, Obesity, Cyanotic Heart Disease
Dysrhythmia	A-V Block, Post Cardiac Surgery Cardiomyopathy
High Blood Pressure	H.T., Coarctation, Obesity
Hyperglycemia and Ketoacidosis	IDDM (Insulin Deprivation)
Hypoglycemia	IDDM
"Ischemic" ST-T	Aortic Stenosis and Insufficiency Mitral Prolapse, Coarctation, Sickle-Cell Anemia
O2 Desaturation	C.F., Cyanotic H.D.
Seizures	Epilepsy
Syncope	A-V Block, Aortic Stenosis

Safe exercise for the child with asthma

The main deleterious effect of exercise in the child with asthma is the well documented exercise-induced asthma (EIA) which, under certain conditions, would occur in the great majority of patients (Shephard, 1977). Although no long-term cure of EIA is available, there are several means of preventing its occurrence during or following an exercise bout. These are listed in Table 2.

Table 2: Means of preventing or ameliorating exercise-induced asthma

1. Preventing the cooling or drying of airways
– Reduce activities in cold/dry climate
– Emphasize water-based activities
– Use face mask or scarf
– Try nasal breathing

2. Utilizing the refractory period
– Perform a preliminary activity before main activity
– Intensity and duration of preliminary activity to be determined individually

3. Using medications
– Inhaled beta2 agonist is the drug of choice
– Sodium chromoglycate is a secondary line of defence
– Try inhaled steroids or ipratropium bromide if the above are inadequate

4. Other means
– Reduce exercise intensity when asthma is uncontrolled
– Aerobic training may increase the intensity threshold for EIA

Minimize airway cooling or drying

One strategy of preventing EIA is based on the protective nature of humid or warm inspired air, compared with dry or cool air (Bar-Or et al., 1977; Chen & Horton, 1977; Deal et al., 1979; Hahn et al., 1984). One possible recommendation is to reduce the intensity and duration of PA when weather is cold or dry. This approach, however, may markedly restrict outdoor activities of asthmatic residents of cold climatic regions.

Alternative approaches are to reduce the cooling or drying of the airway during exercise. One of these would be to emphasize aquatic activities, because of the high water content of the air close to water level. Indeed, the partial protective effect of high humidity of inspired air during swimming has been documented in children with asthma (Bar-Yishay et al., 1982). Another means of humidifying and warming the air before it reaches the airways is by covering the mouth with a scarf or surgical-like face mask. A pocket of air is created between the face and the mask or the scarf. This pocket traps some of the expired air, which is mixed with the inspired air of the next breath. The resulting added dead space is apparently too small to interfere with the child's alveolar gas exchange. Indeed, as shown by

Brenner et al. (1980) and by Schachter et al. (1981), wearing a mask markedly reduced the bronchoconstrictive effect of exercise. Finally, warming and humidification of the inspired air can be achieved when the child inhales through the nose, rather than through the mouth (Proctor, 1977). Indeed, when patients with asthma used nasal breathing during treadmill exercise (Shturman-Ellstein et al., 1978) or free running (Mangla & Menon, 1981), their airways showed considerably less bronchoconstriction than when they inhaled through their mouth. The practicality of this approach is limited, however, to mild intensities of exercise, when ventilatory volume is low. At higher volumes, nasal breathing causes a high resistance to air flow, which is incompatible with the increased ventilatory demands during moderate to intense exertion.

Utilize the refractory period

When a patient with asthma performs two consecutive bouts of exercise within a period of up to 2-3 hours the second bout will often not induce asthma, or the intensity of asthma will be lower than that induced by the first bout. The period following the first exercise bout, during which the patient is fully or partially protected has been termed "refractory period" (Edmunds et al., 1978). One suggested mechanism for such refractoriness is that the first bout of exercise induces a release of prostaglandins, particularly PGE-2, which protect the airways from subsequent constriction (O'Byrne & Jones, 1986; Wilson et al., 1994). Such a release takes place following the first bout, irrespective of whether that bout induced EIA or not (Ben-Dov et al., 1982; Wilson & Bar-Or, 1989; Wilson et al., 1990). The practical implication is that refractoriness can be achieved without prior EIA. Another practical question is how intense should the first bout be in order to induce refractoriness. Data from one study (Wilson & Bar-Or, 1989) suggest two patterns of response: In some patients the initial bout has to be intense (yielding a heart rate of 170 beat/min), In order to induce appreciable refractoriness. In others, however, there seems to be no relationship between the intensity of bout 1 and the degree of refractoriness that it produces. There is a third group of patients (nearly 50% of those who respond to exercise with EIA) who show no protection following bout 1, irrespective of its intensity.

Patients, coaches and physical educators should become familiar with the phenomenon of refractory period because, with the choice of a suitable warm-up (that would trigger refractoriness), the patient can be protected from EIA during or following the actual competition or practice session. Because of the inter-individual variability in the degree of response, patients should be tested at various intensities of bout 1, in order to determine their pattern of response.

More research is needed to determine the intra-individual consistency in achieving refractoriness, to identify optimal warming-up regimens for various activities and to determine why only some of the patients with asthma exhibit refractoriness to EIA.

Use medications

Several medications have been found suitable for the prevention or amelioration of EIA. This presentation is not intended to provide a comprehensive review of this therapeutic approach. For further details, see Morton & Fitch (1992). Before any medication is considered for EIA, one must make sure that the child's asthma is under control. Inhaled beta-2 agonists are usually recognized as the first line of defence. Their advantage over other agents is that they act within minutes and, as such, can be taken just prior to the activity. In addition, a beta-2 agonist such as Ventolin can be used to stop an attack of EIA once it has started. Cromolyn (disodium cromoglycate) is another potent agent for prevention of EIA, but it does not stop an attack once it has started. If neither of these agents (or both combined) helps, then one should consider an inhaled steroid, taken on a chronic basis, or an anticholinergic agent, such as ipratropium bromide.

It is seldom that competitive athletes with asthma can practice or compete successfully without the help of a medication. However, for the non-athletic population one should first consider the use of other means of managing EIA.

Reduce the exercise intensity

For most patients, EIA is exercise-intensity dependent: It seldom occurs before exercise has reached a moderate-to-high intensity (e.g., 60% maximal O_2 uptake or more) (Wilson & Evans, 1981). This is why standardized exercise provocation tests for EIA are held at heart rates of at least 160-170 beat/min. The physiological basis for such a threshold phenomenon is that minute ventilation, together with the temperature and humidity of inspired air, determines the degree of airways cooling or drying which, in turn, determines the degree of EIA.

A practical implication of the above phenomenon might be that patients should adopt activities of mild to moderate intensities. This, however, is unsuitable for children and youth who participate in competitive sports and for many others whose less structured, spontaneous activities call for high-intensity exertion. A recommendation to avoid intense activities should therefore be limited to patients with severe asthma, who do not respond to other means of preventing EIA.

Increase the aerobic fitness

A question often asked is whether improvement of physical fitness can be used as a mean of reducing EIA. Some authors (e.g., Bundgaard, 1989; Oseid & Haaland, 1978; Svenonius et al., 1983), but not all (Fitch et al., 1976; Mitsubayashi, 1984), found that an aerobic training program induced a reduction in the severity of EIA. Only one of the quoted studies (Bundgaard, 1989) included randomly assigned controls, so the issue is still open for more definitive experiments. If indeed aerobic training causes a reduction in the severity and prevalence of EIA the mechanism is, most probably, through a reduction in minute ventilation at any given submaximal exercise intensity, rather than a specific effect on the development of EIA.

From a practical point of view, asthma is not a contraindication for training at any intensity. Patients with asthma can excel in sports and reach world class levels. For the non-athletic child with asthma, the best prescribed activity is swimming (Bar-Or & Inbar, 1992), or other water-based sports. This is not merely because of the lower asthmogenicity of such sports, as discussed above. Swimming training has been shown to induce specific clinical benefits to children with asthma, such as reduction in morbidity, better school attendance and a lower reliance on medications (Huang et al., 1989).

Safe exercise for the child with cystic fibrosis

The two abnormal responses to exercise in patients with CF are arterial O_2 desaturation and dehydration. The latter may lead to heat-related disorders.

Oxygen desaturation

O_2 desaturation occurs during maximal or near-maximal exercise intensities (Cerny & Armitage, 1989), mostly in patients with an advanced disease (Neijens, 1989). Common wisdom suggests that such patients should be instructed to avoid intense activities. There is, however, no evidence that exercising while the arterial O_2 content is depressed presents any danger to the child with CF. Furthermore, it is possible that, because of O_2 desaturation, the child has a limited ability to sustain high-intensity aerobic activities and, thus, will spontaneously limit his or her activities when reaching marked O_2 desaturation. More research is needed to study this important issue.

Voluntary dehydration and its prevention

Children with CF have a poor heat tolerance, and their morbidity and mortality increase during climatic heat waves (Kessler & Anderson, 1951). As recently shown (Bar-Or et al., 1992), children with CF who exercise in a hot environment drink less and, as a result, dehydrate excessively compared with healthy children. Furthermore, even several hours following a prolonged race their drinking volume is still insufficient to fully replenish prior fluid losses (Stanghelle & Skyberg, 1988).

An increase in osmolality of the extracellular fluid is a major trigger for thirst, through activation of hypothalamic osmoreceptors. This process normally occurs in people who perspire, because of the hypotonic ionic concentration of their sweat (and a resulting increase in body fluid osmolality). The insufficient voluntary drinking of patients with CF is, most probably, due to the extremely high concentration of NaCl in their sweat, which moderates the increase in body fluid osmolality and dampens their thirst drive. The end result is that children with CF, who exercise in the heat, gradually dehydrate, even when drinking water is provided to them *ad libitum* (Bar-Or et al., 1992). The resulting "voluntary dehydration" is, most likely, the cause for their heat intolerance.

In the above experiment, the fluid presented to the children was unflavoured water. In a recent study with healthy children who exercised intermittently at 35°C, 50% relative humidity for three hours (Wilk & Bar-Or, in press), voluntary drinking volume increased by 44% when the subjects were given flavoured water, instead of unflavoured water. The drinking volume increased further (additional 45%) when the children were given a flavoured salt (NaCl), (18.8 mmol x l^{-1}) and carbohydrate (6%) solution. These findings strongly suggest the importance of NaCl in enhancing thirst, which may be an effective means of preventing voluntary dehydration in patients with CF. An experimental confirmation of this hypothesis is currently underway in the author's laboratory.

Safe exercise for the child with insulin-dependent diabetes mellitus

The main deleterious response to prolonged exercise in patients with IDDM is hypoglycemia. A much less common disorder is exercise-induce hyperglycemia and ketoacidosis, which may occur when the patient is deprived of insulin.

Hypoglycemia and its prevention

Exercise-induced hypoglycemia may occur during activities that last 30 minutes or more, in patients who are well insulinized. It reflects a higher utilization of glucose, mostly by the active muscles, than its production by the liver. This is mediated through an increase, sometimes uncontrolled, of insulin release from the injection site, as well as through an increase in the sensitivity of insulin receptors (Dorchy, 1996). A recent study (McNiven et al., 1995) suggested a high test-retest reliability of the blood lowering effect of moderate-intensity exercise in children or adolescents with IDDM. The study also showed that these patients could not subjectively gauge their blood glucose levels during prolonged exercise, until they reached a hypoglycemic range.

Textbook approaches to the prevention of exercise-induced hypoglycemia include: Decreasing (by 10 to 50%) the insulin dose, choosing injection sites for insulin over muscle groups that are less likely to participate in a given exercise (e.g., upper arm in a cyclist), and increasing the carbohydrate consumption during and prior to exercise. The latter recommendation does not address differences in carbohydrate needs, based on the amount of exercise or on body mass (see, for example, Kistler, 1995).

An attempt has been made by this author (Bar-Or, 1983) to quantify the recommended carbohydrate intake, based on the calculated amount of glucose utilized during various physical activities and sports. The assumption was that, during fairly intense activities, 60% of the energy sources is derived on the average from carbohydrates. These recommendations, however, were based on several assumptions and on extrapolation from adults-based tables of energy expenditure, rather than on experimental evidence.

In a current project in our laboratory, adolescents with IDDM were given on two occasions an identical exercise protocol of 2x30 min cycling at 60% of predetermined maximal O_2 uptake. Their blood glucose was monitored periodically prior to, during and following the exercise. The two visits differed in the beverage provided to the subjects. In visit 1 they drank plain water. In visit 2 they were given an 8% carbohydrate solution. Total carbohydrate quantity equalled its utilization by each subject, as determined from the O_2 uptake and respiratory exchange ratio during visit 1. The carbohydrate solution in visit 2 was enriched by ^{13}C isotope and measurement of the $^{13}C/^{12}C$ ratio in the expired air allowed to determine how much of the exogenous carbohydrate was utilized during the one-hour exercise. Preliminary results suggest that, while the protocol of visit 1 was accompanied by a consistent reduction in blood glucose levels, this drop was almost abolished during visit 2, even though only 14% of the exogenous carbohydrate was oxidized in that visit. The above data suggest that, when simple carbohydrates are given as a drink to patients with a well controlled IDDM, in a quantity equal to glucose utilization, exercise-induced hypoglycemia can be prevented. More research is needed to find out whether the above is true in patients whose diabetes is not well controlled. One should also study the effects of complex carbohydrates, presented as solids or solutions, on the glycemic response to exercise.

Hyperglycemia & ketoacidosis and its prevention

When a patient with IDDM is insulin deprived, glucose production by the liver is enhanced, without a concomitant increase in its assimilation to the exercising muscles (Dorchy et al., 1977). As shown experimentally (Berger et al., 1977), the above combination may induce hyperglycemia and ketoacidosis in the exercising adult with IDDM. Even though there are no similar experiments with children and adolescents, one should assume that they will incur the same deleterious response. Thus, to be on the safe side, a child with IDDM who is under-insulinized should not be allowed to perform physical activities.

Challenges for future research

Understanding the pathogenesis of any deleterious effect of exercise is a key to its prevention. For example: Why do children with cyanotic heart disease perspire excessively (and are thus prone to dehydration)? what is the reason that exercise may induce a crisis in sickle cell anemia? if, indeed, exertion causes damage to the muscle fibres of a child with Duchenne muscular dystrophy, what is the mechanism?

Another area that requires further knowledge is *how enhanced physical activity interacts with other therapeutic modalities*, such as medications or diet. For example, how much adjustment in insulin dosage is required in order to attain safe exercise for the child with IDDM? should one adjust, based on the level of physical activity, steroid dosage in a child with hypophyseal insufficiency, or the anticonvulsant medication in a child with epilepsy?

For ethical reasons, *one should not conduct intervention studies with children, where the end point is damage* (e.g., stress fractures in a child who has developed osteopenia following therapy for leukemia, or a heat stroke in a child with CF who has reached high degree of hypohydration). One alternative is to keep a long-term, multi-centre registry of such mishaps and accidents. This, using sound epidemiological principles, will allow to document the actual incidence of detrimental effects of exertion in children with a chronic disease.

References

Barber, G. Training and the pediatric patient: a cardiologist's perspective. In: Blimkie, C.J.R., and O. Bar-Or (eds.) New Horizons in Pediatric Exercise Science. Champaign, IL: Human Kinetics, 1995, pp. 137-146.

Bar-Or, O. Pediatric Sports Medicine for the Practitioner. From Physiologic Principles to Clinical Applications. New York: Springer Verlag, 1983.

Bar-Or, O., and T. Baranowski. Physical activity, adiposity and obesity among adolescents. Pediatr. Exerc. Sci. 6: 348-360, 1994.

Bar-Or, O., C.J.R. Blimkie, J.A. Hay, J.D. MacDougall, D.S. Ward, and W.M. Wilson. Voluntary dehydration and heat intolerance in cystic fibrosis. The Lancet 339:696-699, 1992.

Bar-Or, O. and O. Inbar. Swimming and asthma: Benefits and deleterious effects. Sports Med. 14:397-405, 1992.

Bar-Or, O., I. Neuman, and R. Dotan. Effect of dry and humid climates on exercise-induced asthma in children and pre-adolescents. J. Allergy Clin. Immunol. 69:163-167, 1977.

Bar-Yishay E, I. Gur, O. Inbar, I Neuman, R.A. Dlin, and S. Godfrey. Differences between swimming and running as stimuli for exercise-induced asthma. Europ. J. Appl. Physiol. 48: 387-397, 1982.

Ben-Dov, I., E. Bar-Yishay, and S. Godfrey. Refractory period after exercise-induced asthma unexplained by respiratory heat loss. Am. Rev. Resp. Dis. 125: 53-534, 1982.

Berger M, P. Berchtold, H.-J. Cuppers, H. Drost, H.K. Kley, W.A. Muller, W. Wiegelmann, H. Zimmermann-Telschow, F.A. Gries, H.L. Kruskemper, and H. Zimmermann. Metabolic and hormonal effects of muscular exercise in juvenile type diabetics. Diabetologia 13:355-365, 1977.

Brenner, A., P. Weiser, K. Krogh, and M. Loren. Effectiveness of a portable face mask in attenuating exercise-induced asthma. J. Am. Med. Ass. 244: 2196-2198, 1980.

Bundgaard A: Physical training in bronchial asthma. Scand. J. Sports Sci. 10:97-105, 1989.

Cerny F.J., L.M. Armitage. Exercise and cystic fibrosis: a review. Pediatr. Exerc. Sci. 1:116-126, 1989.

Chen, W.Y., and D.J. Horton. Heat and water loss from the airways and exercise-induced asthma. Respiration 34: 305-313, 1977.

Deal, E.C. Jr., E.R., Jr. McFadden, R.H. Jr. Ingram, and J.J. Jaeger. Hyperpnea and heat flux: initial reaction sequence in exercise-induced asthma. J. Appl. Physiol: Resp. Environ. Exerc. Physiol. 46: 476-483, 1979.

Dlin, R. Adolescent hypertension and sports. In: Bar-Or, O. (ed.). Encyclopedia of Sports Medicine. Vol. 6: The Child and Adolescent Athlete, Oxford: Blackwell Scientific, 1996, pp. 480-492.

Dorchy, H., G. Niset, H. Ooms, J.R. Poortmans, and D. Baran. Study of the coefficient of glucose assimilation during muscular exercise in diabetic adolescents deprived of insulin. Diabète Métab. (Paris) 3: 31-34, 1977.

Dorchy, H., and J.R. Poortmans. Juvenile diabetes and sports. In: Bar-Or, O. (ed.). Encyclopedia of Sports Medicine. Vol. 6: The Child and Adolescent Athlete, Oxford: Blackwell Scientific, 1996, pp. 455-479.

Edmunds, A.T., M. Tooley, and S. Godfrey. The refractory period after exercise-induced asthma: Its duration and relation to the intensity of exercise. Am. Rev. Resp. Dis. 117: 247-254, 1978.

Fitch K., R.A. Morton, and B.A. Blanksby. Effects of swimming training on children with asthma. Arch. Dis. Child. 51: 190-194, 1976.

Hahn, A., S.A. Anderson, A. Morton, J. Black, and K.A. Fitch. Reinterpretation of the effect of temperature and water content of the inspired air in exercise-induced asthma. Am. Rev. Resp. Dis. 130: 575-579, 1984.

Huang S.W., R. Veiga, U. Sila, E. Reed, and S. Hines. The effect of swimming in asthmatic children – participants in a swimming program in the city of Baltimore. J. Asthma 26: 117-121, 1989.

Kessler, W.R., and D.H. Anderson. Heat prostration in fibrocystic disease of the pancreas and other conditions. Pediatrics 8: 648-656, 1951.

Kistler, J. Children and adolescents. In: Ruderman, N., and J.T Devlin (eds.). The Health Professional's Guide to Diabetes and Exercise. Alexandria, VA, American Diabets Association, 1995, pp. 218-222.

Mangla, P.K., and M.P.S. Menon. Effect of nasal and oral breathing on exercise-induced asthma. Clin. Allergy 11: 433-439, 1981.

McNiven, M.Y., O. Bar-Or, and M. Riddell. The reliability and repeatability of the blood glucose response to prolonged exercise in adolescent males with insulin-dependent diabetes mellitus. Diabetes Care 18: 326-332, 1995.

Mitsubayashi T. Effect of physical training on exercise-induced bronchospasm of institutionalized asthmatic children. Arerugi 33: 318-327, 1984

Morton, A., and K. Fitch. Asthmatic drugs and competitive sports. An update. Sports Med. 14:228-242, 1992.

Neijens H.J. Exercise and the child with bronchial asthma. In: Bar-Or O, ed. Advances in Pediatric Sport Sciences. Champaign, Ill: Human Kinetics, 1989, pp. 191-201.

O'Byrne, P.M., and G.L. Jones. The effects of indomethacin on exercise-induced bronchoconstriction and refractoriness after exercise. Am. Rev. Resp. Dis. 134: 69-72, 1986.

Orenstein, D.M. Asthma and sports. In: Bar-Or, O. (ed.). Encyclopedia of Sports Medicine. Vol. 6: The Child and Adolescent Athlete, Oxford: Blackwell Scientific, 1996, pp. 433-454.

Oseid, S., and K. Haaland. Exercise studies on asthmatic children before and after physical training. In: Eriksson B., and B. Furberg (eds.) Swimming Medicine IV. Baltimore: University Park Press, 1978, pp. 32-41.

Perrault, H. Benefits of exercise training after surgical repair of congenital heart disease. A theoretical perspective. In Blimkie, C.J.R., and O. Bar-Or (eds.) New Horizons in Pediatric Exercise Science. Champaign, IL: Human Kinetics, 1995, pp. 123-135.

Proctor, D.F. The upper airways. Nasal physiology and defense of the lungs. Am. Rev Resp. Dis. 115: 97-129, 1977.

Schachter, E., E. Lach, & M. Lee. The protective effect of a cold weather mask on exercise-induced asthma. Ann. Allergy 46: 12-16, 1981.

Shephard, R.J. Exercise-induced bronchospasm – a review. Med. Sci. Sports 9: 1-10, 1977.

Shturman-Ellstein,R.J. Zeballos, J.M. Buckley, and J.F. Souhrada. The beneficial effect of nasal breathing on exercise-induced bronchoconstriction. Am. Rev. Resp. Dis. 118: 65-73, 1978.

Stanghelle, J.K, and D. Skyberg. Cystic fibrosis patients running in marathon. Int. J. Sports Med. 9(suppl):37-40, 1988.

Steadward, R.D., and G.D. Wheeler. The young athlete with a motor disability. In: Bar-Or, O. (ed.). Encyclopedia of Sports Medicine. Vol. 6: The Child and Adolescent Athlete, Oxford: Blackwell Scientific, 1996, pp. 493-520.

Svenonius E., R. Kautto, and M. Arborelius. Improvement after training of children with exercise-induced asthma. Acta Paediatr. Scand. 72: 23-30, 1983.

Wilk, B., and O. Bar-Or. Effect of drink flavor and NaCl on voluntary drinking and rehydration in boys exercising in the heat. J. Appl. Physiology. In press.

Wilson, B.A. and O. Bar-Or. Refractoriness to exercise-induced bronchoconstriction and the intensity of prior exercise. Med. Sci. Sports Exerc. 21:S21, 1989.

Wilson, B.A., O. Bar-Or, and P.M. O'Byrne. The effects of indomethacin on refractoriness following exercise both with and without a bronchoconstrictor response. Eur. Respir. J. 7: 2174-2176, 1994.

Wilson, B.A., O. Bar-Or, and L.G. Seed. Effects of humid air breathing during arm or tread-mill exercise on exercise-induced bronchoconstriction and refractoriness. Am. Rev. Respir. Dis. y142:349-352, 1990.

Wilson, B.A., and J.N. Evans. Standardization of work intensity for evaluation of exercise-induced bronchoconstriction. Europ. J. Appl. Physiol. 47: 289-294, 1981.

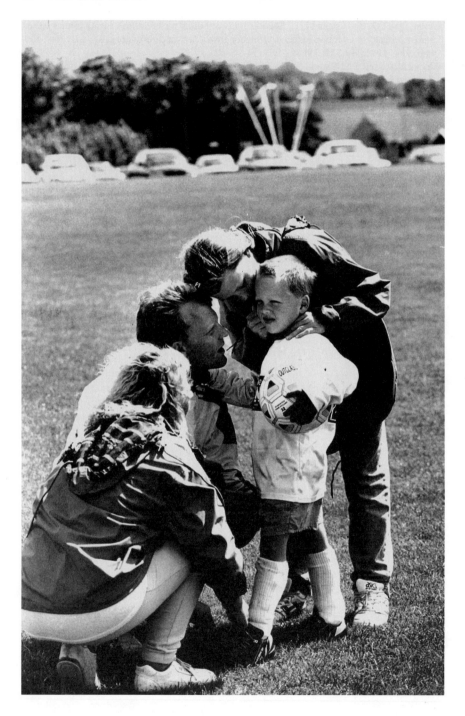

Chapter 2

The Future of Pediatric Exercise Sciences

Per-Olof Åstrand

Physiology, a dying discipline?

A first and very pertinent question is "what is the future of physiology?". That question was asked by Pinter and Pinter in an article in News in Physiological Scinces (NIPS) published in 1993. I am also inspired by an article written by my good friend Björn Folkow, also published in NIPS in 1994. In 1987 the past president of the American Physiological Society, Howard E. Morgan wrote in Physiological Reviews (1987): "Physiology is an integrative science that has as its goal discovering the mechanisms of overall bodily function and its regulation. The types of data to be integrated are wide ranging and include studies at the following levels: cellular and molecular, whole organ and tissue, and whole animal. All of these pieces of information are needed to provide a comprehensive understanding of basic mechanisms and their regulation. As an extension of this view, the research approach that is taken should not impact on the ability of the physiologist to teach a broad-based course in human physiology to medical students. Those physiologists who work at the systems level must be fully aware of advances at the cellular and molecular level, whereas those who work on molecular mechanisms must be able to integrate their data into a model of systemic function."

What is the situation today? Folkow (1994) points out that throughout history fads and fashions have strongly influenced human beliefs and activities, ranging from political systems to women's hats. Scientists and thereby science, are not immune to such trends, which sometimes have accelerated but not seldomly rather retarded or distorted progress. In biomedical research the latest justifiable enthusiasm, has emerged from the great methodological developments in molecular biology that have revolutionized genetics, microbiology, cell biology, and so forth.

However, such surges of success within some sectors of biomedical research have also had dangerous consequences. In this particular case they have fascinated the scientific community to the extent that in the long run perhaps even more important aspects of life sciences threaten to be neglected. After all, above the cellular level comes the infinitely more complex hierarchies of function and control that characterize higher organisms, with *Homo sapiens sapiens* topping the list thanks to their neocortical abilities.

Folkow (1994) emphasizes that some leaders of physiology departments, being thus expected spokespersons in their faculties for the integrative physiology have been so carried away by the popular molecular-cellular bandwagon as to more or less vanish below the cell membrane, bringing most co-workers with them in the deep dive, presumably never to emerge again. Some even seem to be ashamed of their noble discipline, which made men like Ludwig, Bernard, Starling, Cannon and Wiggers proud of the profession with traditions back to William Harvey. Thus they often try to find new names for their departments, spiced with "in" words such as *molecular* and *cellular*. Furthermore, as became evident at the teaching session of the Centennial Helsinki Congress of the International Union of Physiological Sciences (IUPS) in 1989, some physiological departments are no longer competent to provide their medical students with an acceptable course concerning the function of humans, e.g. during physical activity in various environments.

In the mentioned article by Pinter and Pinter they write: "While in 1982 and 1986 broadly interpreted integrative (or organ, or systems) physiology had 90-95% share of the total research support given by the United States National Institutes of Health to physiological departments of US medical schools. In 1991 this share among the five top recipients had diminished to an average of 70% of the total and was down to 30% of research funds in one prominent institution. Even more indicative are figures tabulated by members of the Association of Chairmen of Departments of Physiology. According to this source, for in-training programs, across the board only 16% of both pre- and postdoctoral participants received systems approach training in their preparation for a career in physiology. It is difficult to see how 84% of the young physiologists entering the profession would be able to cope with the task of instructing medical students."

Folkow uses a rough parallel. The present trend bears some resemblance to an imagined situation in which the board of directors of the Boeing or Douglas jumbojet industries become so fascinated by the production of microchips and similar minicomponents that they forget to hire aerodynamic experts and feedback specialists, not to mention test pilots. Soon they would end up with mountains of sophisticated junk, but certainly they would be without airplanes that could fly. He quotes a statement by an old producer of building bricks who, on joining a tourist trip to Rome and confronting the magnificent splendor and gigantic vaults of Michelangelo's St. Peter's dome, dryly remarked, "trivialities, compared with brick production."

Fortunately, the tide may have started to turn, at long last. For example, the American Physiological Society (APS) has, via its long-range planning committee, presented an important report concerning "the future of physiology", published under the telling Shakespearean title, "What's Past is Prologue" (1990). While molecular biology has often been called "the new biology" the APS committee sums up: "integrative biology – the biology of the future."

At the recent IUPS Congress in Glasgow, 1993, with, as honorary presidents, five British Nobel laureates in physiology or medicine, integrative physiology was made the leading theme. In a way, this is best illustrated by the following 1992 quotation on physiology and the future from *Physiological Society Magazine*, where the ideas behind the Congress and its planning were discussed:

"It is a major challenge, for the end of the 20th century sees physiological science benefiting from an unprecedented wealth of information at the cellular and molecular levels. The "black boxes" discovered by cell biophysics (ion conductance, pumps, carriers) have been opened by molecular biological techniques, while intracellular events are probed in great detail by fluorescent and other indicators. The great intellectual challenge now is to start to reintegrate this information into an understanding of whole tissues, organs, and organisms."

In the June (1994) issue of the *Physiologist* signed by approximately 700 esteemed physiologists addressed to the US congress there is an emphasize on the essential role of integrative biomedical sciences in protecting and contributing to the health and well-being of the nation.

To sum up, for a physiologist it is a pleasure to qoute Starling: "The physiology of today is the medicine of tomorrow." In my opinion, exercise physiology is from these viewpoints particularly important because an exercise situation in various environments provides a unique opportunity to study how different functions are regulated and integrated. It brings the lifeless pieces of molecular and cellular biology into living systems. In fact, most functions and structures are in one way or the other affected by acute and chronic (i.e., in a training program) exercises. Also adaptation to a high altitude or hot environment are other examples of demands of integrative approaches. So, exercise physiology is to a high degree an integrated science that has as its goal the revelation of the mechanisms of overall bodily function and its regulation. It is regretable that so few pages in standard textbooks in physiology for medical students are devoted to discussions of the effects of exercise on different functions and structures. That may explain why a majority of physicians do not spontaneously recommend habitual physical activity. After this introduction, over to pediatrics.

Biological versus chronological age

Since maturation age differs markedly, it is positive that research on adolescents more and more try to relate data to biological age as a baseline, e.g. to age at Peak Height Velocity (PHV-age). That is particularly important in longitudinal studies. Certainly one problem is that one can not in advance predict when a child will reach PHV-age,

In Gunilla Lindgren's study (1978), PHV-age occured as early as at age 9.5 yr for some girls, but not until 15 yr for others. In boys the range was from 11 to 17 yr. At chronological age 13 yr we can find a boy with a weight of 30 kg and a height of 130 cm, and his classmate may weigh 80 kg and be 180 cm tall. It is a challenge to be a physical education teacher: how to avoid accidents, e.g. in contact sports, how to stimulate the small pupil whose physical performances will inevitably be inferior to the large classmate. The "early bird" may dominate in some sports due to the advantages of increased body height, muscle mass, and aerobic power. Additionally the early maturing child, coach, and parents are happy because big money may wait around the corner. However, peers with real talent for a specific sport may catch up, and eventually pass the early maturer. The "early bird" missed that talent and there is a risk that she/he, disappointed, loses interest in sports. What kind of educational principles can be applied to teach 9-10 year old girls and boys about consequences of large variation in maturitional age? In the long run, a late PHV-age may not impose any biological handicap but there may be psychological problems.

To divide young participants in sport events according to chronological age is traditional and very practical but it is very unbiological, and therefore unfair. However, I have no alternative to suggest. It is an interesting observation that in soccer, among teenagers, a majority are born early in the year (Brewer et al., 1995). In my opinion competition in marathons should be prohibited until some years after PHV-age. Then again, we are facing the large range in that age. One solution could be to choose average PHV-age plus 2-3 standard deviations.

It is still debated whether high intensity and volume training may affect PHV-age and timing of menarche. Malina after a review of the literature concludes that in the vast majority of athletes, intensive training for sports has no effect on growth and maturational processes. Menarche is to a higher extent affected by biological selective factors and social factors (Malina, 1994).

Health aspects

There is an unanimous agreement among health educators that young people should, for an optimal development get involved in regular physical activity. Therefore they should be encouraged to adopt such a life style and sustain it into and during adult life. From that point of view it is sad that politicians and administrators in industrialized countries gradually reduce the time alotted for compulsary physical education in schools' curriculum. In the UK, the Department for Education advises that schools provide a minimum of two hours for physical exercise a week, yet a study published in March 1995 showed that the number of state schools where pupils are getting less than this amount has doubled since 1987 (Smith, 1995). In Sweden there has been a quite dramatic reduction in time for physical education in schools over the last decades.

There are positive reports: Engström (1990) found in Sweden that between 1968 and 1984 there was an impressive increase in the percentage of 15-year-olds who belong to sport clubs; the percentage for boys increased from 50% to 70%, and for girls from 17% to 50%. The sad part of the story is that the total number of active young people had diminished. The explanation is that in 1984 almost none was involved in sports during leisure time unless they were members of sport clubs. Therefore, compulsory physical education in the school is essential.

In their recent review, Riddoch and Boreham (1995) point out that the amount and type of physical activity undertaken during childhood that is appropriate for optimal health is unknown, although it has been suggested that, in the absence of such criteria, activity levels known to confer health benefits in adults are also appropriate for children. These authors also report that there are studies in the US and UK indicating that over 69% of children 12 years of age have at least 1 modifiable risk factor for coronary heart disease (CHD). Unfavourable blood lipid and lipo-protein profiles are common during childhood and adolescence and about 13% of young people can be classified as "overweight" (Armstrong, 1995). Thus, there is a trend that the number of overweight young people increases.

One interesting area of research is the question whether there are future health gains when girls during adolescence invest in a "bone bank" by weight-bearing and muscle-strengthening activities, thereby increasing the bone mass. Slemenda et al.(1991) showed a consistent positive association between physical activity and bone density in 118 children aged 5-14 yr.

Prepubertal children appear to be capable of responding to endurance training with improvements in maximal aerobic power. Such adaptations are qualitatively similar, but probably quantitatively less compared with those in adults (Rowland, 1992). There is a similar effect with training of muscle strength. Endurance training has a possible therapeutic value in common diseases of childhood such as asthma, cerebral palsy, cystic fibrosis, diabetes mellitus, hypertension, myopa-thies, and obesity (for references see Schober, 1995). As mentioned, there is a definite trend that children and adolescents are more obese now than decades ago, and reduced physical activity can be one explanatory factor. Body fatness is a risk factor for several diseases (Williams et al., 1992). The question is what is the op-timal intensity, frequency, and duration of the programs we would like to recom-mend? We will face medical and ethical problem: As time goes by research in genetics will reveal more and more defect genes signaling risks for specific diseases. Should efforts be made to search for defect genes already in childhood? The problem is that there will probably be a long gap before one learns about chances to prevent or delay an appearence of the disease. A second question is whether the disease is inevitable, what are the influences of environmental factors including habitual physical activity?

According to the WHO approximately 30% of all people with disabilities are children. Definitely pediatric exercise physiology has an important role in efforts to prevent accidents, and to improve rehabilitation programs.

In a recent review Viru and Smirnova (1995) discuss health promotion and exercise training. Haskell (1994) argues that quantity and quality of exercise to obtain health-related benefits may differ from what is recommended for physical fitness benefits. He points out that the view taken by advocates of the physical activity-health paradigm is that for many people, especially those inclined not to perform more vigorous exercise, and they are in majority, some benefit is better than none. "The greatest health benefits from an increase in physical activity appear to occur when very sedentary persons begin a regular program of moder-ate intensity, endurance type activity. Further increases in intensity or amount of activity appear to produce further benefits in some, but not all, biological or clinical parameters. The magnitude of benefits becomes less for a similar increase in intensity and/or amount of activity" (Haskell, 1994). At a recent meeting in Stockholm, the message was that close to 70% of total medical costs are spent on preventable diseases. This discussion is mainly based on studies on adults but is probably also relevant for children and adolescents. In their review Riddoch and Boreham (1995) point out that we need better data regarding what constitutes a healthy level of physical activity for children in terms of both the quantity and the nature of the activity. Such data may only result from longitudinal studies of children, monitoring health-related behaviours such as physical activity, and observing health outcomes in adulthood. The problem is that those who start such longitudinal studies must believe in personal long lives! Malina (1994) points out that there is no prospective work that can link, with any degree of certainty, health in adult years with childhood activity pattern. The curriculum in physical education is quite different in different countries, but the drop in participation in physical activity after high school/college is relatively universal. Therefore, the key factor behind reduced physical activity is probably not the experiences during lectures in physical education but simply a consequence of human nature. Children have an "appetite center" for physical activity in games, and play. Unfortunately we as adults too often shout "Can't you keep quite!" instead of securing and inspiring a place where they can play. At the symposium it was emphasized that the physical education sports should be adapted to the youngsters and not the kids to the sports!

Motor control

Of importance for motor control is vision, vestibular organ, and the proprioceptors. These systems are well developed early in life, but they are not fully integrated until the age of approximately 8 yr, certainly with individual variation. We know very little about whether specific activities can positively affect this integration. I know teachers who claim that children with difficulties in reading and writing can reduce these handicaps by specific activities, but I have not seen any scientific support for such beneficial effects. Extra attention may be the essential part of the claimed success. Research is needed.

How to find talent for sport?

Above it was emphasized that it is important to separate the discussion of optimal physical activity for health reasons and well-being on one hand and improved fitness on the other. Children spontaneously try their skill, strength, speed, and most of them like to compete. The balancing act is to prevent "too much" for those youngsters who have talent for competitive sports. There are risks for trauma, especially before and during puberty, e.g. injuries to the epiphysical plate of the bones in the legs. It is recommended that training should be supervised by experienced medical expertise. There is a need for education of parents, coaches, and teachers. Particularly former East Germany was an example for successful scouting for young talent and very efficient training. However, there are some clouds over some of the successes. It is interesting to note that in the Olympic Games in Seoul in 1988 female swimmers from East Germany took 10 out of 15 gold medals, but males only 1. In the Olympic games in Barcelona in 1992 German female swimmers only won 1 of the 15 gold medals, male swimmers none.

In this context it should be mentioned that in Sweden, in 1985, we had 5 tennis players who were ranked among the top 15 players in the world. They were active in many sports before age 14, at which age they started to specialize in tennis. They were compared with a group of players who were as good or better at tennis when 12 to 14 yr old. These players specialized much earlier in tennis, trained more, and matured earlier. Therefore they performed well but apparently they were not gifted enough to reach world class (Carlson, 1988). It is best if children and young teenagers try many sports; they should taste a "smörgåsbord" of events, and they should not concentrate on one event until after PHV-age. One conclusion from the mentioned study is that performance at age 12 to 14 yr is not a good predictor of future elite achievements. Malina (1990) pointed out that with few exeptions, inter-age correlations for indicators of growth, fitness, and cardiovascular status are generally moderate to low and thus have limited predictive utility.

Stress testing

When I collected data for my thesis on 141 girls and boys, age from 4 up to 18 yr, published in 1952, I noticed that in many of them it was not possible to establish a "levelling off" of oxygen uptake when increasing the speed of treadmill until the intensity was reached, which exhausted the subjects in 4 to 6 minutes. The measurements were spread over a period of a few weeks. This finding has been confirmed. A second criteria for evaluation of a "maximal" effort was a high peak lactate concentration in blood sampled during early recovery. I would like more cautiousness when authors publish "maximal" data on oxygen uptake, heart rate, lactate concentration, and pulmonary ventilation during exercise. Age predicted maximal heart rate is useless in this connection because one standard deviation is 10 beats x min^{-1} or higher. I also caution against prediction of maximal oxygen uptake from data obtained at submaximal exercise or the quite popular 20 m shuttle run and "Beep-test". I have observed authors who conclude that the shuttle run test is a good predictor of this maximum based on a correlation coefficient being below 0.7. Even when much higher, around 0.9, a closer look at the data may reveal that measured maximal oxygen uptake of, say 2.8 l x min^{-1}, includes predicted values from 2.5 up to 3.4 l x min^{-1}. Data collected on growing individuals often cover a large range which may secure a high correlation coefficient but a large standard deviation is unfortunately not considered.

Summary

There is a definite demand for research on health promoting physical activity in children and adolescents. There is too much of extrapolation from data obtained on adults. Longitudinal studies are important. One problem is the ethical limitations in experiments and "manipulations" of young people including sociology, nutrition, and chemical substances, not to mention commercial aspects. What should we teach pupils, teachers, politicians, administrators? Will it be possible in near future to provide a consensus report/program based on hard scientific data for the minimal/optimal time, volume, intensity for physical education in the curriculum, with special emphasis on improvement in endurance, sprints, strength, motor skills, specific events, leisure time activities to promote health for different ages, including gender aspects? I doubt it. Particularly since at one stage one must consider biological age. It has been pointed out that the relationship between habitual physical activity and health related fitness is very complex. Many of the sport events popular at young ages have a short life span, like American football, soccer, basketball, ice hockey, and track and field events. Realistic recreational sports for future activities like many racket sports, golf, orienteering, swimming, non-sophisticated, individually adapted "aerobics", strength training programs are not without complications to include in the curriculum, particularly considering less time and economical support allotted to programs in compulsory physical education in schools.

I have, maybe, a naive hope that a renewed interest in the school system should be devoted to teaching biology, including insects, e.g. butterflies, and flowers, mushrooms, bird watching, education and thereby interest in the environment and the milieu. Quite a few people do not enjoy going out for a walk because it is recommended for health benefits, but they do accept it "happily" if it is part of a hobby.

References

Armstrong N. Keynote speech: Children, physical activity and health. In: FJ Ring (ed.). Children in Sport. Centre for Continuing Education, University of Bath, Avon. 1995, 5-16.
Brewer J, Balsom P, Davis J. Seasonal birth distribution amongst European soccer players. Sports Exercise and Injury. 1:154-157, 1995.
Carlson R. The socialization of elite tennis players in Sweden: An analysis of the players' backgrounds and development, Sociology of Sport Journal. 5:241-256, 1988.
Engström LM. Sports activities among young people in Sweden – trends and changes. In: R Telema, L Laakso, M Piéron I Ruoppila, V Vihko (eds.). Physical Activity and Life-long physical Activity. Report of Physical Culture and Health, Jyväskylä 73. 1990, 11-23.
Folkow B. Increasing importance of integrative physiology in the era of molecular biology. News in Physiological Sciences. 9:93-95, 1994.
Haskell WL. Health consequences of physical activity: Understanding and challenges regarding dose-response. Med Sci Sports Exerc. 26:649-660, 1994.
Lindgren G. Growth of school children with early, average and late ages of peak height velocity. Ann Human Biol. 5:253-267, 1978.
Malina RM. Physical growth and biological maturation of young athletes. Exercise and Sport Sciences Reviews, 22:389-434, 1994.
Pinter G, Pinter V. Is physiology a dying discipline? News in Physiological Sciences. 8:94-95, 1993.
Riddoch CJ, Boreham AG. The health-related physical activity of children. Sports Med. 19(2):86-102, 1995.
Rowland TW. Aerobic responses to physical training in children. In: RJ Shephard, P-O Åstrand (eds.). Endurance in Sports. Blackwell Scientific Publications, London. 1992, 381-389.
Schober P. Effectiveness of endurance training in children. In: FJ Ring (ed.) Children in Sport. Centre for Continuing Education, University of Bath, Avon. 1995, 101-113.
Slemenda SW, Miller JZ, Hui SL, Reister TK, Johnston CC. Role of physical activity in the development of skeletal mass in children. J Bone Min Research. 6:1227-1233, 1991.
Smith K. Inquiry into Provisions of Physical Education in Schools 1994, Aylesbury Grammar School, March 1995.
Viru A, Smirnova T. Health promotion and exercise training. Sports Med. 19(2):123-136, 1995.

Williams D, Going S, Lohman T, et al. Body fatness and risk for elevated blood pressure, total cholesterol, and serum lipoprotein ratios in children and adolescents. Am J Public Health. 82:358-363, 1992.

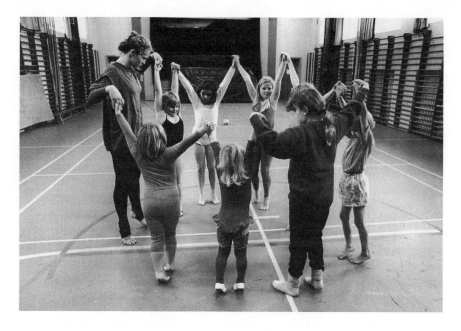

Chapter 3

Genetic and Environmental Factors Related to the Development of Obesity in Youngsters

Thorkild I.A. Sørensen

Genetic epidemiology

When studying genetic and environmental factors it should be kept in mind that:

- Genes and environment are involved in all biological processes.
- Human beings share the genes and the environment that make them different from other species.
- Differences between human beings may be due to different genes, different environment or both.
- Genes work only by being expressed into proteins which immediately interact with the environment.

Being interested in public health and preventive medicine why study the genes if the aim is to get knowledge that can be used to prevent disease? Prevention of diseases requires modification of the contributing causal factors, and genes cannot be modified or eliminated outside the discipline of clinical genetics, where genetic counseling, induced abortion, and gene therapy may be used. The answer is that the study of genes and environment provides better understanding of disease causation, better prediction of disease risk, and better assesment of environmental factors. We may get rid of some of the biases and confounding in the study of disease causation, and have a better view of effect-modification. Eventually, we may get access to modifiable factors that influence gene expression.

This perspective is the basis for the rather new discipline of genetic epidemiology, which may be defined as *'The study of the interplay of genes and environment in the origin of disease.'* The discipline approaches disease causation as an integrated factor without giving priority to genes over environment, or environment over genes.

Environmental influences

Obesity is, as expected, strongly influenced by the environment (1). There is a tendency to consider either genes or environment as the cause of obesity, but both contribute. Influence by the environment is proven by the changes in occurence of obesity over time within populations and within individuals, and changes in occurence by environmental manipulation in populations, in clinical settings and in laboratory experiments.

Familial aggregation

On the other hand, obesity shows a distinct and well established familial aggregation in all populations studied so far (2). The familial aggregation may be due to the genes shared by descent, shared exposure to environmental factors, or a combination of the two. The basic research questions in genetic epidemiology are:

– To what extent can the familial correlations be attributed to the shared genes, or the shared exposure to environmental factors?
– Does shared exposure to environmental factors contribute to the familial correlation after the rearing family environment is left?
– What are the contributions of genetic differences to the interindividual, within-population differences in human fatness? This is actually the heritability question.

There are three separate strategies for addressing the contribution of genes and environment: the nuclear or natural family study, the adoption study, the twin study, and various combinations of these strategies.

Twin studies

In an American twin study from Virginia, 10-11 years old children had their sub-scapular skinfold, triceps skinfold, subiliac skinfold and body mass index (BMI) measured (2). The correlation in these measures among the monozygotic twins were about twice the correlations among the dizygotic-twins, suggesting that all the within-twin similarity is explained by the genes. There are several reservations to be made regarding the twin method, but this will not be dealt with here.

Adoption studies

A complementary method for addressing the basic questions is the study of adoptees (2), which we had a chance to do here in Denmark. The basis for the adoption study design is that adoptees share their genes with the biological family and their family environment with the adoptive family, which allows disentangling the effect of the genes and the environment. Correlations in traits and risk of diseases of adoptees within biological families is assumed to be due to shared genes. Correlations in traits and risk of disease of adoptees in the adoptive family is due to shared family environment.

It is feasible to expand the parent-offspring pedigrees by use of the population registers in our country, for example, by including biological full siblings and paternal or maternal half siblings of the adoptees. There may be various types of adoptive sibs as well, who share family environment with the adoptees, but no genes.

It is neccessary to make a distinction between complete and partial adoption studies (2). The complete ones are those where we have access to the information on the biological family. In such studies the resemblance of the adoptee and the members of the biological family suggest effects of shared genes. Resemblance of the adoptee and members of the adoptive family suggest shared exposure to the same environmental factors. Resemblance may be measured by the correlations of the phenotypes.

In the partial adoption method, the biological families are unavailable for the study. As in the complete adoption study, the resemblance of the adoptee and the members of the adoptive family is due to shared exposure to environmental factors. The resemblance of the members of natural families reflect the combined effects of shared genes and shared exposure to environmental factors. The natural family that is used for comparison can be the biologically related member of the adoptive family or a quite different set of natural families. The genetic effect is then measured by subtraction of the familial environmental effects from the total familial effects. The critique of this method is that the genetic effects are indirectly estimated.

There are three complete adoption studies of obesity (2): the Danish study that was initiated by an American, Dr. Stunkard, and in which I have been involved (3-6), and two American studies conducted in Iowa and Colorado. There are more partial adoption studies beginning with Withers' study in London in 1964 and then several American and Canadian studies (2).

The Danish adoption study

The following presents in more detail, the study that we have conducted with a particular focus on childhood (3-6). By mailed questionaires we obtained height and weight on a population of 3,500 adult adoptees. We then selected four groups: thin, medium weight, overweight, and obese groups, identified their biological and adoptive parents, and asked them or their children about their BMI. The BMI of the parents increased by adoptee weight group, supporting that genes contribute to the familial aggregation. We were quite surprised to see that the BMI of the adoptive father and mother showed no relationship at all to the adoptee weight group. Thus, there appears to be no persistent effects on BMI of the family environment, and all familial aggregation among adults may therefore be attributed to genetic influence (3).

We also looked at the BMI of the biological siblings, i.e. the full siblings, the maternal half siblings, and the paternal half siblings (4). We again have the BMI and the four groups of thin, medium, overweight and obese. For the full siblings, there was a very clear trend in BMI across the adoptee weight groups, even stronger than for the parents. Although we would not expect the same for the half siblings because they share on average only a quarter of the genes, we did see a trend, slightly stronger for the maternal than for the paternal half siblings.

The correlation between the BMI of the biological mother and the adoptees was about 0.15, clearly significant. The correlations between BMI of the biological mother and her other children, the full siblings and the maternal half siblings of the adoptees, were about the same, as expected if family environment has no persisting effect. The correlations with the father were a little more unstable, but showed a similar pattern.

The correlations between the adoptees and the biological full siblings, who have been seperated from the beginning of their lives, were about 0.2, which is slightly lower than in usual family studies, probably because of attenuation of the correlations due to errors in the self-reported measures. The correlation between biological siblings who have been together during childhood are at the same level as the correlations with the adoptees.

When all this is included in a comprehensive, complex path model, the only factor that links these phenotypes is the genetic effects (5). The model included a variety of intra familial environmental effects, which all were non-significant. The model produced a heritability estimate of 34%, which is also at the level of other family studies. Since there were no familial environmental effects, this result indicates that 66%, apart from measurement errors, is due to influences of the non-shared family environment.

Genetic and environmental effects in childhood

To estimate the genetic and familial environmental effects in childhood (6), we found the records of the school health examination for the selected adoptees and their biological and adoptive siblings who grew up in the Copenhagen municipality. The correlation in BMI from 7 to adulthood, from 8 to adulthood etc, showed a stable tracking correlation at the level of 0.35 for all types of relatives.

The correlations between BMI of the biological mother and her offspring during school age were about the same level of the adult correlations, and clearly significant. The correlations between adoptees and their biological full-siblings through this age range were quite high, but they compare well with the correlations among natural siblings.

The correlations between the adoptee and the adoptive mother were much lower, and barely significant. Even lower correlations were found for the adoptive father. The correlations between the adoptees and the adoptive siblings were somewhat unstable; some of them were significant, but they were obviously less than those between biological full siblings and adoptees. Taken together, the results indicate that there may be an effect of the shared environment on the BMI in childhood.

From this adoption study, we conclude that the genetic influences on the BMI are already expressed by the age of seven at the same level as in adulthood. The rearing environment as shaped by the mother appears to have a weak influence.

We may speculate that the very high correlations between the biologically related siblings is due to non additive genetic transmission, possibly by major recessive genes. Furthermore, if the heritability is stable over time, implying stable geno-type-phenotype correlations, then the genetic influence may explain the tracking of BMI from childhood through adult life.

If all the adoption studies are put together (2), we see quite a heterogeneuos pattern of results for the partial studies, but a clear and consistent pattern for the complete studies, all emphasizing the genetic influence. So, concluding from these studies, we may say that all the complete and some of the partial adoption studies indicate that the familial resemblance in fatness from childhood to adulthood is mainly due to shared genes. All the complete and some of the partial studies found little or no influence of shared family environment, particularly after the adoptee had left the home. In view of the differences in design and strength, it is fair to put more emphasis on the evidence from the complete studies.

Major gene effects

1994 an exciting development in the search for the major genes possibly underlying these genetic effects has begun with the identification and sequencing of the mouse OB gene and the human homologue OB gene by J.R. Friedman's group (7). Even though we are working with a quantative trait, such as BMI, it makes sense to identify sub populations within this distribution that may be influenced in terms of their position in the distribution by specific genes (2). So called segregation analysis of the distribution of BMI within natural families have suggested that there may be major gene effect underlying this continuous distribution, but, of course, it is quite indirect evidence.

Several genes are supposed to be associated with obesity, but so far none of the candidate genes have shown any consistent link in human studies (2). Some mutations of the OB gene may cause excessive obesity in mice, but the first studies examining variations in this gene in human populations do not support its role in human obesity.

Gene-environment interaction

There is some evidence suggesting gene-environment interaction in human obesity. So called commingling analysis of the BMI distribution among monozygotic twins suggests a combination of a major gene with gene-environment interaction (8). The combined two-dimensional distribution of BMI of the monozygotic twins can be separated into one that is quite narrow within the range of the central, the most normal, part of the BMI distribution, and a flat and broader one at a higher BMI. This may be interpreted as follows: a major gene may cause some of the twins to be susceptible to environmental influences producing obesity, and this group constitutes the upper part of the BMI distribution, where the correlation is lower than in the central part because of the variation in environmental influences.

This is also the message from the very famous and very carefully conducted experimental study by our colleague, Dr. Claude Bouchard and his group at Laval University in Canada (9). A sample of monozygotic twins went through 100 days of strict regulation of dietary intake, and the changes in body weight and body composition were measured. The correlation between twins in changes in body weight is surprisingly low. Since measurement errors and departures from the experimental design can be considered very small, this result suggests that the preceding, accumulated environmental effect has a strong influence on the response to the diet. The within-pair similarity as well as the between pair differences may be attributed to identity of the genes within the twin pairs and differences in genes between the pairs, causing the pairs to respond differently to the same environmental exposure – the experimental diet. However, effects due to preceding, accumulated environmental influences shared by twin pairs, but being different between these pairs must be kept in mind as a possible alternative interpretation.

Further evidence of gene-environment interaction comes from a 6-year follow-up study of a population of women from Gothenburg, Sweden (10), where dietary fat intake was related to later changes in BMI. The women and their parents were grouped according to overweight. Only the group who had excessive fat intake, were overweight and had overweight parents, showed an increase in BMI. This suggests that subjects with this familial predisposition – which according to the adoption and twin studies is a genetic predisposition – are sensitive to excessive fat intake.

Secular trends in obesity

This section provides an explanation of some secular trend studies that we have conducted in Denmark (1). Young men examined at the draft boards from 1943 until 1974 showed a prevalence of extreme overweight, defined as BMI exceeding 31, that was quite stable until about 1960. Thereafter, the prevalence of extreme overweight rose steeply. While this occurred, the central part of the distribution, indicated by the median level, was stable throughout the time period.

Can this be explained by the changes in fat intake? The dietary fat consumption on the society level increased a few years before the rise in prevalence of extreme overweight (11). This suggests that the increased fat intake by a particular subset of the population with a particular genetic susceptibility led to the increasing prevalence of obesity.

We have seen similar secular trends in Danish boys born between 1930 and 1965, whose height and weight have been measured at the annual health examinations in the schools of the Copenhagen municipality. We have computerized about 146,000 growth charts from these birth cohorts. The median BMI at age 7 was very stable over the 36 years. Also the lower part of the distribution was very stable, but in the upper part of the distribution there was a clear increase. The same pattern is seen at all ages up age 13 years.

In the draftee studies, the rise in prevalence began at year of birth 1942 (1). During the stable period at the beginning of 1930 the prevalence was about 1 per 1000, corresponding to the 99.9 percentile. We defined extreme overweight among the boys born between 1930 and 1934 by the 99.9 percentile of the BMI, and applied this criterion to the remainder of the school boy population. The increasing trend in extreme overweight among the boys also began in 1940-1942. So, we conclude from those analyses that there was a stable central part of the BMI distribution, corresponding to the range between the 1st and 80th percentiles, with a progressive increase in the right tail over this time period in the birth cohort 1930 to 1965 of Danish boys aged 7 to 13 years. This increase in extreme overweight is parallel to the increase among the Danish young men. We may hypothesize that these trends reflect a gene-environment interaction, where a subset of the population carrying a specific major gene is more susceptible to the rise in fat intake.

Energy balance determinants

There is experimental, clinical and epidemiological evidence suggesting that decreased physical activity may also play a causal role in obesity. Body mass, body fat and body energy is influenced by a biological and behavioral interplay, and nutritient partitioning is an important issue related to accumulation of fat as well as to energy expenditure (2). We typically think that accumulation of fat must be the result of an excess intake relative to expenditure, which of course is true in terms of the descriptive physico-chemical relationship. What is creating it, is the important question. It can be a primary increase in energy intake, or it can be a primary decrease in energy expenditure, but it can also be due to a primary tendency to accumulate fat, which then would indirectly create the energy imbalance.

Future research

Future research should address the following issues:

- More accurate measures of the size and distribution of fat mass.
- Assessment of gender and age-related genetic effects.
- Assessment of non-additive genetic effects.
- Characterization of the familial environmental influences.
- Assessment of gene-environment interactions, including the role of physical activity.
- Assessment of physiological and biochemical mediators.
- Identification of the genes responsible for the genetic effect not least for the gene-environment interactions.

References

1. Sonne-Holm S, Sørensen TIA. Post-war course of the prevalence of extreme overweight among Danish young men. J Chron Dis 1977;30:351-8.
2. Bouchard C (ed). The Genetics of Obesity. Boca Raton, CRC Press: 1994.
3. Stunkard AJ, Sørensen TIA, Hanis C, Teasdale TW, Chakraborty R, Schull WJ, Schulsinger F. An adoption study of human obesity. N Engl J Med 1986;314:193-8.
4. Sørensen TIA, Price RA, Stunkard AJ, Schulsinger F. Genetics of obesity in adult adoptees and their biological siblings. BMJ 1989;298:87-90.

5. Vogler GP, Sørensen TIA, Stunkard AJ, Srinivasan MR, Rao DC. Influence of genes and shared family environment on adult body mass index assessed in an adoption study by a comprehensive path model. Int J Obes 1995;19:40-5.
6. Sørensen TIA, Holst C, Stunkard AJ. Childhood body mass index – genetic and familial environmental influences assessed in a longitudinal adoption study. Int J Obesity 1992;16:705-14.
7. Zhang Y, Proenca R, Maffei M, Barone M, Leopold L, Friedman JM. Positional cloning of the mouse obese gene and its human homologue. Nature 1994;372:425-32.
8. Price RA, Stunkard AJ. Commingling analysis of obesity in twins. Hum Hered 1989;39:121-35.
9. Bouchard C, Tremblay A, Després JP, Nadeu A, Lupien PJ, Thériault G, Dussault J, Moorjani S, Pinault S, Fournier G.. The response to long-term overfeeding in identical twins. N Engl J Med 1990;322:1477-82.
10. Heitmann BL, Lissner L, Sørensen TIA, Bengtsson C. Dietary fat intake and weight gain in women genetically predisposed for obesity. Am J Clin Nutr 1995;61:1213-7
11. Lissner L, Heitmann BL. Review: Dietary fat and obesity: evidence from epidemiology. Eur J Clin Nutr 1995;49:79-90.

Questions

Q1:   What was the criterea for being thin, medium, and overweight and obese?

TIAS: In the adoption study of the adults, the thin ones were those who were below the age- and gender-specific fourth percentile, the medium were the four percent around the median, the obese were the four percent in the top, and the overweight were the four percent next to the obese. Given the size of total population from which we selected the adoptees there is no doubt about the thinness of the thin group, and those who were in the obese group had a BMI above 30 or so.

Q1:   Did you measure body fat content just from skinfolds, or only by the BMI?

TIAS: In the adoption studies of the adults we have self-reported weight and height, and in childhood it was measured height and weight in schools. We used an additional measure, namely body silhouette scores ranging from the very thin to the very obese and this gave about the same results. But this is admittedly a weak part of the study and I think that in the future we need to measure body composition, for example using bioimpedance technique.

Q1:   Were you not conserned with the potential for misclassification of overweight having used only the measure of BMI, since someone with a high muscular mass will likely have a high BMI, despite relatively low body fast mass?

TIAS: Sure, this is a classical problem in obesity epidemiology. There seems to be a quite good correlation, however, between BMI and measures of body fat, particularly in the extremes of the distribution.

Q2:   I think it is very fortunate to have this large resource of children going back to 1930 to look at the secular trends. But one thing that surprises me is that during the Second World War, the level was very flat compared with the data from Holland, where there was extensive, nutritional restriction. I wonder if you have any comment on that?

TIAS: You are probably referring to the exciting Dutch famine study. In Denmark, there was no famine during the war. We were actually still producing a lot of food. I would be reluctant to associate the change in 1942 or around the early 1940s to anything that has to do with the war, because it was persistent for a long time after the war. Also, it is of course very exciting that the increase in obesity prevalence, or at least part of it, seems to be cohort specific. Those born in 1942 constitute the first birth cohort, which makes one think that it is some very early exposures that are relevant. There is a very exciting and slightly provocative coincidence here: In 1942 visits by public health nurses to the mothers and their newborns to give the mother advice about how to feed the child (among other things) became a general service.

Q3:   I was interested in your emphasis on the higher end of the scale, the very obese. Is there any evidence that you know of for a threshold on health effects or even some hint of a threshold on health effects?

TIAS: There are numerous very large studies about the health effects of BMI, millions of peoples followed for many years. I think it is fair to say that if you stick to one measurement of BMI in adulthood you begin to see increased mortality and increased detrimental health effects when you exceed a BMI of 25 and it becomes obvious when you are at a BMI of 30. Now the new and very important aspect is that the distribution of fat on the body, particularly the amount of visceral fat seems to be a major carrier of the effect on mortality and health of the increase in BMI. If, in these large populations we could seperate the size of the visceral fat from the remaining body fat, we might see that the visceral fat explains most if not all of the detrimental effects. Of course, if you are morbidly obese, there are a lot of other effects than what comes from the visceral fat. One of the recent recommendations from our British colleagues about how to deal with obesity on a public health level is not to measure height and weight, but to measure the abdominal circumference as a measure of visceral fat as a more appropriate target of intervention.

Q4:   In the last 10-15 years, a tremendous increase in critical obesity in the British population has taken place with an increase from 5% to 12%. Over the same period, there has been a drop in calorie intake, and the increase in obesity nicely matches the decrease in physical activity, the increase in car-ownership, and the increase in television watching.

TIAS: This substantiates what we have seen in Denmark, and we have some new data suggesting that the increase in prevalence of obesity has continued. Next I think that both fat intake and physical activity are important, but not necessarily total calorie intake. From the physiological point of view, the combination of the relative amount of fat in the diet and the physical activity is what matters. So, if you are physically inactive and combine this with a relatively high dietary fat intake, then you are at high risk, and this high risk may be partially genetically determined. It has been argued that since obesity is so frequent, genes are not really what we should look for. My suggestion will be that if you understand the genetic interaction, then we may be better off in terms of designing interventions and setting up precise actions against this trend.

Q5:   I am from Holland and born in 1941. I was interested in your data looking at the increase in fat intake or the percentage of the dietary intake of fat and obesity. You have already mentioned it, but it is not a general finding that it is the fat intake that makes you fat. It can also be the carbohydrate and the proteins. Do you have the same contribution for the other components?

TIAS: There seems to be a lack of very good prospective studies that can seperate these effects. The matter is also complicated by the fact that there is an automatic link between the amount of fat and the amount of carbohydrate, given quite a stable protein intake. An overview of the cross-sectional studies and the few prospective studies suggests that there is evidence for the importance of fat intake (11). The physiologists tell me that there is no evidence to support that carbohydrate, even with excessive intake, is converted into fat in the humans.

Q6:   The concept of BMI may be simple, but I have some problems really understanding the use of BMI as an expression of overweight. It is defined as weight divided by height to the second power. If you apply a dimensional analysis, weight is the same as body volume multiplied by the average body density. So BMI then should be proportional to height to the third, divided by height to the second power, that is proportional to height. You should have a higher BMI the fatter you are. So why then can we apply BMI values in general and without making any distinction between people, for example between children and adults. The same applies to the secular trend in body height. Could an increase in body height explain the increases in BMI?

TIAS: First of all, the BMI as far as I see it, is a good index from a very pragmatic point of view in terms of providing an empirical basis to remove the height dependency of weight. So, you can just iterate what is the optimal power of height that removes the correlation between height and the index, and this is very close to two; in some studies of women it is lower and in some younger ages it is a bit higher than two, but among young men and I think through most of childhood it works very well. But I know that Alex Roche has done a very careful study of the feasibility and validity of the BMI as a measure and has some generalizations to suggest. Would you like to help me answering this question?

Alex Roche: I do not think we ought to exaggerate the importance of BMI, but it is useful. And I think in determining whether it is useful you can use several criteria. One is that there are a lot of data around for weight and for stature, much more than there are for waist circumference, and they exist in retrospective data sets such as the childrens' study that you are going to do around the schools. So there is a case for using weight and stature. How should you then combine weight and stature? You can do it in terms of saying that you want an index of obesity and you want and index that is highly correlated with weight and is independent of stature. And then you will, as Thorkild said, come up with powers of stature that are not necessarily two, but are very close to two. If you think now, I do not really want it to be correlated with weight and independent of stature because why should it be. Really I would rather have an index that is highly correlated with percent body fat. Then all these indices, whether you talk about relative weight or weight over stature squared, or weight over stature cubed, or weight to the one third power over stature, they have all got very similar correlations with the same body fat, so it does not really matter very much. One advantage of weight over stature squared is that there is extensive literature about it, relating BMI to morbidity and to mortality. This is a reason to hang on to it for the time being. The other thing that you can do is to maximize the relationship between weight and stature and percent body fat by giving fractional powers to weight and to stature, and we did that at one stage. We came up with weight to power 1.2 over stature to the power 3.3, but our relationship with percent body fat was no better than the relationship of BMI with the same body fat. So there are a lot of practical reasons to stay with the BMI. The other point I would like to make is this: do not go back to relative weight. Relative weight is disasterous, because it relates to the reference data that you are using. So, relative weight of 110% or 120%, which has been used as an index for overweight, or as an index of obesity, is determined by the reference data that you use, and this is not the way the body works. The body does not know which reference data that you use. The body works in relation to, how much weight you have for the stature that you have, not to where you are in relation to a set of reference data.

TIAS: I may add to this that we have assessed whether the secular trends were the same in the short and the tall Danish young men and the results were the same. The rise in extreme overweight is totally height independent among the draftees.

Q7:   Your paper is about what happens on a population level. On an individual level there is another set of variables, which reflect how the individual reacts to that environment. The same environment can have different inter relationships to the environment in the family. For eating behaviour you may get a disconnection in the normal satiety mechanism so that eating is no longer driven by a sense of hunger and satiety, but often as emotional eating. Television may have a double effect: not only are you inactive watching TV, but there is also the visual stimulus. The question is whether you have some neuropsychologically interacting stimulation even to eat more while you watch television. The emotional feelings of either anger, depression and boredom often lead to more eating. So I wonder if on that individual level we will see this disconnection from normal physiology. Will you comment on that?

TIAS: I completely agree that we have to take into account this complexity when we move from the statement of familial environment to a more specific description of what is the familial environment. Even within the family, the environment may not be familial. It may be specific for the individual, and this will be reflected by the way that we analyse the data. So what is called shared family environment here, is what can possible be attributed to what is shared. I fully agree with the necessity of incorporating psychological mechanisms and possible neuro-endocrinological mechanisms here. We have conducted another study on school children, independent from the one presented here, where we had a chance to follow about 800 school children for whom information was gathered from their teacher about how their parents were caring for them, and independent of the teacher, from the school nurse. The teacher was just stating whether he/she had the impression that the parents were interested in what was happening to the child, with neglect at the bottom of the scale. From the school nurse we got information about this kind of parental attention, namely if the child appeared dirty and poorly groomed. This gave us two measures of poor parental care compared to usual expectations. Those who were at the bottom of these two scales were at greatly increased risk of becoming obese ten years later, when a follow-up was made. Even when we controlled for other relevant variables, such as socio-economic variables and BMI at the time of entry, we found the same risk. Whether the parental neglect is genetic or environmental within the family or family context, we do not know.

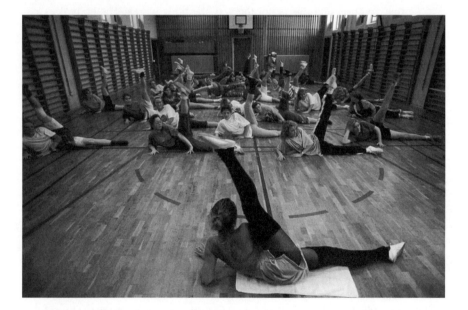

Chapter 4

Growth and Hormone Release in Children and Adolescents: Are they Altered by Athletic Training?

James N. Roemmich, Pamela A. Clark and Alan D. Rogol

Introduction

Continued physiological growth of a child is generally considered a sign of health and well-being. How a child fits in with his/her peers can be derived from comparison of an individual with a normal group as represented by the percentile lines on a growth chart. These are based on cross-sectional data derived from the measurement of many children at various ages. However, individual children do not necessarily grow according to these standard curves, and a *longitudinal* growth chart derived from the growth points of the *same* child over *time* more accurately defines the growth pattern of any individual child. By definition, normal (physiological) growth encompasses the 95% confidence interval for the specific population in question. Most children and adolescents with a normal growth pattern, but who remain below the lower 2.5 percentile (approximately -2.0 SD), will be otherwise normal. The further below the -2.0 SD mark, the more likely that the individual has a condition that is keeping him/her from reaching the genetically-determined height potential.

Normal growth

Linear growth velocity rapidly decelerates from approximately 30 cm x year^{-1} during the first few months of life to approximately 9 cm x year^{-1} at 2 years to 7 cm x year^{-1} at age 5 years. Size at birth is determined by the intrauterine environment as well as by genetic (polygenic) factors. Between birth and approximately 2 years of age infants make adjustments for these maternal factors and increase or decrease their linear growth velocity in relationship to the norm to reach their genetically determined growth potential. Linear growth then continues at approximately 5.5 cm x year^{-1} until puberty is imminent. At that time there is a gradual slowing ("preadolescent dip"), before the onset of the pubertal growth spurt.

For an average girl, the growth velocity increases sharply at approximately 10 years of age, reaches a peak of approximately 10.5 cm x year^{-1} at 12 years and then decelerates toward zero as bone epiphyseal closure ensues around the age of 15 years. For boys who follow the average curve, the pubertal growth spurt begins around the age of 12 years, reaches a peak velocity of 12 cm x year^{-1} at the age of 14 and then decelerates toward zero around the age of 17 years. The total growth at puberty averages approximately 25 cm for girls and 28 cm for boys. If one takes into account the 2 additional years of prepubertal growth for boys one can account for the 13 cm (5+5+3) difference in the mean adult height between men and women.

Any single point on the growth chart is not very informative. When several growth points are plotted over time, it should become apparent whether that individual's growth is average, a variant of the norm or pathologic (growth failure). The point at which an individual is placed at any given time can be related to the *height age*, that age at which that child's height would be at the 50th percentile. It indicates the mean age of children of that measured height in the proper normal population. The height age is determined from the growth chart by drawing a line parallel to the chronological age axis from the child's plotted point to the 50th percentile and then a perpendicular line to the horizontal axis. The intersection of the latter line with the "age" axis is the *height age*.

Normal variants

Normal variants of growth were found in 82% of children whose height fell at the third percentile (-2 SD), but only in 50% of those whose height fell at the first percentile (-3 SD) of the mean for age (Lacey and Parker, 1974). Assessment of skeletal maturation is perhaps the best indicator of biological age or maturity status because its development spans the entire period of growth. There are several methods for determining the former, (Greulich and Pyle, 1959; Roche et al., 1988; Tanner et al., 1983). Each uses a single radiograph of the left hand and wrist and comparison is made to children of normal stature using an atlas and "scoring system." Since girls are more developmentally mature at any given chronological age, separate standards exist for females and males.

Mature height can be predicted based on the midparental height. The adjusted midparental height (target height) is calculated by adding 13 cm (the difference between the 50th percentiles for adult men and women) to the mother's height (for boys) or subtracting 13 cm from the father's height (for girls) and then taking the mean of the height of the same sex parent and the adjusted height of the opposite sex parent. Adding 8.5 cm above and below the midparent target height will approximate the *target height range* of the 3rd to 97th percentile for the anticipated adult height for that child adjusted for his/her midparental stature (genetic potential). Other methods also exist for predicting adult stature of an individual based on mathematical formulations derived from the growth history of that child or from the attained height and bone age of the child as calculated from specific tables.

Familial Short Stature

On average, children of smaller parents will eventually attain lesser height. Children with this condition should grow at an appropriate *rate* during childhood and should attain sexual maturation and the pubertal growth spurt at the usual age since the bone age approximates the chronological age.

Constitutional delay of growth

This variant is considered to be a delay in the *tempo* of growth. Each calendar year is not accompanied by a full year of growth and skeletal development so that the individual requires more time to complete the growth process. Most of the children will eventually have delayed adolescence as well as the delayed attainment of adult stature. The birth history and birth length are generally normal, but the growth pattern shifts downward to the lower percentiles with the lowest values for growth velocity being obtained at approximately three to five years of age. Thereafter, this pattern is characterized by steady progression of growth. Since the bone age does not advance one year for each calendar year it *progressively deviates* from the chronological age. The height age is usually approximately the same as the bone age and, if true, the mature height will be well within the normal range for the appropriate population. This pattern, as for familial short stature, is often familial and since both are relatively common, many children will have elements of both.

Puberty

1. Hormonal control

Puberty is characterized by the onset and continued development of secondary sexual characteristics and an abrupt onset of linear growth (Tanner and Davies, 1985). The secondary sexual characteristics are a result of androgen production from the adrenals in both sexes (adrenarche) and testosterone from the testes in the male and estrogens from the ovaries in the female (gonadarche). The accelerated growth (adolescent growth spurt) derives from the rising levels of the gonadal steroid hormones and also indirectly from increased growth hormone (GH) and insulin-like growth factor I (IGF-I) secretion. The latter hormones are considered the more important (Kerrigan and Rogol, 1992).

Physiological amounts of gonadal steroid hormones alter the neurosecretory activity of the GH producing cells. Boys in late puberty can be distinguished from those earlier in puberty or from young adults by a greater amount of GH release. The physiology of the GH axis (hypothalamus-pituitary-IGF-I) represents a dynamic system that manifests pubertal changes as well as control by multiple neural, hormonal and metabolic influences. The data indicate a major role for gonadal steroid hormone-mediated augmentation of GH at puberty, probably mediated through estrogen-receptor mediated signalling [for review see Kerrigan and Rogol, 1992; and Metzger et al., 1994].

Timing and tempo

The timing and tempo of puberty are predominantly genetically determined. Its onset is characterized by increasing gonadotropin and gonadal steroid hormone secretion. The tempo of puberty, although also genetically determined, does not yet have a defined neuroendocrine mechanism; however, it may be most relevant to the "alterations" in pubertal development considered when studying the impact of strenuous athletic training as well as nutritional aspects on the length and intensity of pubertal development and the attendant increases in linear as well as segmental growth.

Hormonal alterations caused by athletic training

Although alterations in the pulsatile release of GH and LH during athletic training have been reported for adults (Weltman et al., 1992; Rogol et al., 1992), there are no comparable data for children and adolescents. To separate the effects of training, nutrition and normal pubertal process (Kerrigan and Rogol, 1992) would be difficult. Preliminary data from a study of wrestlers noted below indicate a "syndrome" compatible with partial GH insensitivity, based on static measurements of GH, IGF-I and GHBP. Virtually all of the data with regard to the hypothalamic pituitary gonadal axis indicate hypogonadotropic hypogonadism, a state that is physiologic for prepubertal children. Recent data from a group of highly trained swimmers show a condition more closely resembling the pathophysiology of one form of the polycystic ovarian syndrome (hyperandrogenism), but these data await confirmation (Constantini, et al., 1995). In summary, athletes of both sexes may have altered growth and somatic development. With the present data it is difficult to ascribe alterations in the neuroendocrine axes for GH or the gonadotropins as causative. When taken singly or in combination at least the following factors are vital: Genetic selection, volume and intensity or stress of training and competition, macro-and micronutrient sufficiency and the neuroendocrine axes for growth hormone and the gonadotropins.

Effects of physical activity and training on growth and adolescent development

Does physical activity and/or sport training affect linear growth and pubertal maturation? The literature is replete with reports that state that athletic training has salutary, no, or deleterious effects on growth and pubertal development (for review, see Malina, 1994a) However, careful appraisal of the reports often reveals severe methodological faults – lack of consideration of inter-individual variation in biological maturity status and subject selection to name but two factors. Certain sports, especially for males, show advantages to the early maturer and others for girls, especially gymnastics and dance, favor the later developing female. Thus, there is concern about the potential effects of training on the timing and progression (tempo) of puberty "caused" by training and sports participation. Critical analysis using the biological indicators, bone age or peak height velocity in longitudinal study designs, is needed to tease out the effects of such training on pubertal development and mature stature.

Females

Delay in growth and sexual maturation is well documented among certain groups of *elite* female athletes, most notably gymnasts, dancers, and long distance runners (Baxter-Jones, 1994; Claessens, 1992; Lindholm, 1994; Malina 1994b). The underlying mechanisms, however, are not entirely clear, in part due to few longitudinal data in girls. Control of growth and age of menarche involve the complex interaction of a number of factors, including the physical and metabolic demands of intensive athletic training and competition.

Investigations of growth parameters in adolescent female gymnasts consistently find these girls to be shorter and lighter with a significantly lower percentage body fat than age-matched control girls or athletes participating in less strenuous sports such as swimming who generally are taller and mature earlier than normal (Lindholm, 1994; Malina, 1994b; Peltenburg, 1984b; Theintz et al., 1993; Theintz et al., 1994a). Theintz et al (1993) followed a cohort of adolescent gymnasts and swimmers over a 2 to 3 year interval. Training periods averaged 22 hr x wk^{-1} for the gymnasts and 8 hr x wk^{-1} for the swimmers. The gymnasts had significantly lower growth velocities from skeletal age 11 to 13 y, with a peak height velocity of only 5.48 ± 0.32 cm x y^{-1} compared to 8.0 ± 0.50 cm x y^{-1} for the swimmers. Over time height standard deviation scores decreased significantly in the gymnasts, without a change in the chronologic age/bone age ratio. Consequently, predicted heights of the gymnasts decreased with time, but those of the swimmers did not change.

Lindholm et al (1994) also observed slower growth velocities among a group of adolescent female gymnasts. These girls did not display the distinct growth spurt seen in the control group of inactive girls, and 27% had final adult heights less than expected based on parental height predictions. Bernadot et al., (1991) studied 2 groups of female gymnasts, one age 7-10 y and the other 11-14 y. Weight x age^{-1} and height x age^{-1} dropped from the 48th percentile in the younger group to the 20th percentile in the older gymnasts. Body fat did not differ significantly between the age groups, and at all ages the gymnasts had significantly more muscle mass for size.

Several investigations have compared age of menarche among female athletes participating in different sports to the general population. Claessens et al., (1992) found the median age of menarche among a group of gymnasts to be 15.6 ± 2.1 y compared to 13.2 ± 1.2 y for the control population. Theintz et al., (1994a) observed that among a group of gymnasts and swimmers aged 12.7 ± 1.1 y, only 7.4% of the gymnasts had experienced menarche in contrast to 50% of the age-matched swimmers. The gymnasts in this study, however, had a significant delay in skeletal age (-1.42 ± 0.99 y), but the swimmers had comparable chronologic and skeletal ages. This report emphasizes the importance of the interaction between somatic growth and sexual maturation, and the interpretation of physiologically *vs.* pathologically delayed maturation. Baxter-Jones et al (1994) reported the mean ages of menarche among adolescents being intensively trained in gymnastics, swimming, and tennis to be 14.3, 13.3, and 13.2 y, respectively, with a population reference value of 13.0 y. Significant delay was again noted only among the group of gymnasts. The data for gymnasts are replicated to a lesser degree for dancers and runners, and sports such as swimming, speed skating, and tennis appear to have minimal effects on growth or age of menarche (Baxter-Jones, 1994; Malina, 1994a; Malina, 1994b).

Although these data suggest a relationship between intense athletic training and growth and sexual development in gymnasts, the data are not conclusive. When interpreting growth and development data of athletes a host of other variables including the intensity of training must also be considered. An individual's overall state of health is paramount to normal growth and development, but this is assumed to be high in these adolescents who meet the great physical demands of training. Genetic predisposition plays an important role; short stature of gymnasts is often familial (Malina, 1994b; Peltenburg, 1984a) and a positive correlation has been found between menarcheal age in mothers and daughters (Baxter-Jones, 1994; Malina et al., 1993). Historically, socioeconomic class and family size have been influential, with menarche occurring earlier in the higher socioeconomic classes and in families with fewer siblings (Malina, 1983; Tanner, 1989). Psychological and emotional stressors associated with year-long training, frequent competition, maintenance of low body weight, altered peer relationships, and demands of coaches may also influence growth and pubertal timing (Malina, 1994b; Theintz, 1994a).

Nutrition, especially dieting behavior, is a major factor, particularly among sports which emphasize strict weight control. Although the hypothesis of a critical percent body fat (Frisch, 1976) is no longer considered valid, the issue of energy balance is crucial to growth and development. Energy intake, as well as intake of vital nutrients such as calcium necessary for bone accrual, are often suboptimal in athletes who restrict diet during a state of increased metabolic demand. Nutter (1991) found that the desire to be thin may influence dietary patterns of female athletes more than changes in exercise training.

Several investigators have stressed the importance of strenuous physical training *prior* to menarche (Hamilton, 1988; Sidhu, 1980; Theintz, 1994c; Warren, 1980). The younger children may be especially susceptible to the demands of strenuous exercise. Similar trends in type of sport are apparent; however, with menarche in gymnasts more delayed than that in swimmers or tennis players who began training at a comparable age. Prior menstrual irregularity appears to be an important risk factor for oligo/amenorrhea in adolescents who begin training after menarche. Estok et al (1991) evaluated a group of marathon runners, for menstrual history and body composition. Menstrual history proved to be a more important factor than low body fat in the development of oligo/amenorrhea.

Alterations in growth and pubertal maturation are not common among young women engaging in recreational exercise or in those adolescents who train less than 15 hours per week (Bonen, 1992; Theintz, 1994c). The incidence of oligo/amenorrhea and secondary amenorrhea among athletes has been cited as 10-40%, compared to 2-5% for the general population (Hohtari, 1986). The distinction between elite and non-elite athletes is important since it pertains to training time and intensity. Olympic athletes have been shown to have significantly later menarche than high school, college, and club level athletes (Malina et al., 1978; Malina, 1994a). The differing demands of various sports also dictate the amount of time spent in strenuous physical activity; gymnasts and dancers far exceeding swimmers and tennis players in the available studies. Catch-up growth has been reported in gymnasts when training is temporarily reduced or stopped (Theintz, 1994b).

However, one of the most important (perhaps the single most important) variables to take into account is that of *selection bias*. Body types which are most successful are selected for particular sports. Several studies have reported gymnasts to be smaller than peers from a young age (Malina, 1994a; Malina, 1994b; Peltenburg, 1984b). Delayed menarche favors the continuation of sports such as gymnastics, suggesting that elite gymnasts are selected, in part, for this attribute. Continued participation, in turn, leads to more intense training and blurring of cause and effect.

The implications of delayed menarche are directly relevant to the accrual of bone mineral. Since more than 90% of the total adult bone mass is established during the pubertal years, failure to accrue bone mineral at a normal rate during this time may result in permanent deficits. Bone mineralization is a complex process influenced by nutrition (especially calcium intake), weight bearing activity, and the sex steroid hormones. Hypoestrogenism due to pubertal delay or secondary amenorrhea can lead to low bone mineral density despite adequate weight bearing exercise. In a group of female runners Louis et al (1991) found decreases in bone mineral density in all subjects with oligo/amenorrhea, while runners with regular menses had values within the normal range. This has been suggested as one factor contributing to skeletal injuries in gymnasts (Lindholm, 1994).

Males
In general, boys who participate in sport have normal growth rates and are normal or advanced for their state of skeletal and sexual maturation (Malina, 1994a). The advanced states of maturation in athletes may be attributed to the power and performance advantages associated with maturation (Roemmich and Rogol, 1995) which may attract these children to particular sports.

However, for sports that may create an energy drain the effects on growth and maturation are inconclusive. Seefeldt et al., (1988) reported that the height velocity of elite male distance runners was equal to non-running controls during one year of training. Other investigations have reported the growth in height of male distance runners to be either slowed (Daniels and Oldridge, 1971) or advanced (Eriksson, 1972) relative to reference data. Unfortunately, the maturity levels of the runners and/or the reference data were not given for the two former studies so few conclusions can be made drawn with regard to the influence of distance running on growth velocity.

The growth of scholastic wrestlers has also been the concern of several investigations. American wrestlers begin losing weight to certify for lower competitive weight classes as young as 8 years of age (Steen and McKinney, 1986). The weight is lost through dieting, severe exercise, dehydration, and various other methods (Steen and Brownell, 1990) and has produced enough concern to warrant both the American College of Sports Medicine (1976) and American Medical Association (1967) to publish position stands calling for the limitation of this practice. In fact, several authors have speculated that the growth of prepubescent wrestlers may be slowed during the sport-season (Smith 1994; Williams, 1993). As a group, high school wrestlers are usually shorter than the average for their age (Malina, 1994a). However, this is probably a self-selection process for wrestling.

A cross-sectional study compared the growth patterns of 477 high school wrestlers to a representative sample of adolescent males (Housh et al., 1993). The wrestler and reference groups were not different at any age for body weight, but the slope value for the gain in body weight was significantly greater for the reference sample. The reference group was significantly taller than the wrestlers after the age 16.4 years, but the slope values for gain in height were not statistically different. Slope values were also compared for 13 other anthropometric variables with few notable group differences. The investigators concluded that wrestling does not slow growth and maturation. However, the study did not address whether the growth rate during the sport season is slowed and if so, if there is catch-up growth during the off-season.

Several investigations have reported the growth of scholastic wrestlers during and after the sport season. When compared to non-wrestling controls matched for age, maturation and physical characteristics, the growth in height and segmental bone lengths of wrestlers is not decreased during the season or accelerated after (Roemmich, 1994; Roemmich and Sinning 1995, Sinning et al., 1976). The data for breadth measures are less consistent. Investigations have reported both accelerated (Roemmich and Sinning, 1995, Sinning, 1976) and normal (Roemmich, 1994) growth in body breadths during the post-season.

As expected, many investigations have reported reductions in weight, fat mass and percent body fat during the season (Eckerson et al., 1994; Horswill et al., 1990; Hughes, 1991; Roemmich, 1994; Roemmich and Sinning, 1995). However, the fat-free mass is more conserved with most investigators reporting non-significant reductions (Eckerson et al., 1994; Hughes, 1991; Roemmich, 1994; Roemmich and Sinning, 1995), and one reporting a significant decrease (Horswill et al., 1990). Still, the fact that the fat-free mass does not increase as would be expected for normal pubescent males, and that it is related to the loss of arm and leg strength (Roemmich, 1994; Roemmich, Sinning 1995) suggests the statistically non-significant reductions may be *biologically* relevant. After the sport season there is accelerated incremental gains in weight, fat mass, and fat-free mass (Roemmich, 1994; Roemmich and Sinning, 1995; Sinning et al., 1976; Tipton and Tcheng, 1970). The post-season gains in weight can be above the 99 percentile for age (Roemmich, 1994; Roemmich and Sinning, 1995). Accelerated post-seasonal gains in weight, fat mass and fat-free mass suggest soft tissue catch-up growth by the wrestlers. In-season changes in anthropometric measures of lean tissue such as the mid-arm girth and lean limb cross-sectional areas (obtained from skinfold corrected girths), also provide evidence that despite heavy bouts of training, wrestlers can fail to accrue lean tissue during the sport season and show an accelerated accrual during the post-season (Roemmich, 1994; Roemmich and Sinning, 1995).

In summary, there are a few compelling data to implicate training or competition as causal in the shorter stature and decreased body mass in some pubertal athletes in specific sports. What does appear likely is that activities such as gymnastics and dancing in girls or wrestling in boys select for those participants with desirable genetic traits. Added to this process are the interactions among nutrition and the energy drain of training. Preliminary hormonal studies cannot distinguish between constitutionally delayed puberty and a syndrome caused by the sport participation. However, studies designed to make this distinction probably cannot be done in the adolescent group. Investigations in adult women show that some amenorrheic athletes have altered pulsatile gonadotropin release, but it has not yet been possible to separate the impact of the training itself from nutritional and stress factors.

References

American College of Sports Medicine position paper on weight loss in wrestlers. Sports Medicine Bulletin, 1976, 11; 1-2.

American Medical Association position paper on wrestling and weight control. JAMA 1967, 201; 131-133.

Baxter-Jones ADG, Helms P, Baines-Preece J, Preece M. Menarche in intensively trained gymnasts, swimmers and tennis players. Annals of Human Biology 1994; 21:407-415.

Bernadot D, Czerwinski C. Selected body composition and growth measures of junior elite gymnasts. J Amer Dietetic Assoc 1991; 91:29-33.

Bonen A. Recreational exercise does not impair menstrual cycles: A prospective study. Internat J Sports Med 1992; 13:110-120.

Claessens AL, Malina RM, Lefevre J, Beunen G, Stijnen V, Maes H, Veer FM. Growth and menarchal status of elite female gymnasts. Med Sci in Sports Exer 1992; 24:755-763.

Constantini NW, Warren MP. Menstrual dysfunction in swimmers; A distinct entity. JCE&M 1995; 80:2740-2744.

Daniels JT, Oldridge N. Changes in oxygen consumption of young boys during growth and running training. Med Sci in Sports Exer 1971; 3:161-165.

Eckerson JM, Housh DJ, Housh TJ, Johnson GO. Seasonal changes in body composition, strength, and muscular power in high school wrestlers. Ped Exer Sci 1994, 1:39-52.

Eriksson BO. Physical training, oxygen supply and muscle metabolism in 11-13 year old boys. Acta Physiologica Scandinavica 1972, Supplementum 384, 1-48.

Estok PJ, Rudy EB, Just JA. Body-fat measurements and athletic menstrual irregularity. Health Care Women Internat 1991; 12:237-248.

Frisch RE. Fatness of girls from menarche to 18 years, with a nomogram. Hum Biol 1976; 48:353-359.

Greulich WW and Pyle SI. Radiographic atlas of skeletal development of the hand and wrist (2nd ed). Stanford, CA: Stanford University Press, 1959.

Hamilton LH, Brooks-Gunn J, Warren MP, Hamilton WG. The role of selectivity in the pathogenesis of eating problems in ballet dancers. Med Sci Sports Exerc 1988; 20:560-565.

Hohtari H. Effects of Endurance training and season on pituitary-ovarian, -thyroid and -adrenocortical function of female runners and joggers. University of Oulu Printing Center, 1986.

Horswill CA, Park SH, JN Roemmich. Changes in protein nutritional status of adolescent wrestlers. Med Sci Sports Exerc 1990, 22: 599-604.

Housh TJ, Johnson GO, Stout J, Housh DJ. Anthropometric growth patterns of high school wrestlers. Med Sci Sports Exer 1993, 25:1141-1151.

Hughes RA, Housh TJ, Johnson GO. Anthropometric estimations of body composition in wrestlers across a season. J Appl Sport Sci Res 1991, 5:71-76.

Kerrigan JR, Rogol AD. The impact of gonadal steroid hormone action on growth hormone secretion during childhood and adolescence. Endocr Rev 1992;13:281-198.

Lacy KA, Parker JM. The normal short child: Community study of children in Newcastle--upon-Tyne. 1974; 49:417-424.

Lindholm C, Hagenfeldt K, Ringertz BM. Pubertal development in elite juvenile gymnasts. Effects of physical training. Acta Obstet Gynecol Scandinavica 1994, 73:269-273.

Louis O, Demeirleir K, Kalender W, Keizer HA, Platen P, Hollmann W, Osteaux M. Low vertebral bone density values in young non-elite female runners. Internat J Sports Med, 1991; 12:214-217.

Malina RM. Physical activity and training: Effects on stature and the adolescent growth spurt. Med Sci Sports Exerc 1994a, 26:759-766.

Malina RM, Ryan RC, Bonci CM. Age at menarche in athletes, their mothers and sisters. Am J Hum Biol 1993, 5:137.

Malina RM. Physical growth and biological maturation of young athletes. Exer Sport Sci Rev 1994b; 22:389-433.

Malina RM, Spirduso WW, Tate C, Baylor AM. Age at menarche and selected menstrual characteristics in athletes at different competitive levels and in different sports. Med Sci Sports Exer 1978; 10:218-222.

Malina RM. Menarche in athletes: A synthesis and hypothesis. Annals of Hum Biol 1983; 10:1-24.

Metzger DL, Kerrigan JR, Rogol AD. Gonadal steroid hormone regulation of the somatotropic axis during puberty in humans. Trends Endocrinol Metab 1994; 5:290-296.

Nutter J. Seasonal changes in female athletes diets. Int J Sports Nutr 1991; 1:395-407.

Peltenburg AL, Erich WB, Zonderland ML, Bernink MJ, VanDenBrande JL, Huisveld IA. A retrospective growth study of female gymnasts and girl swimmers. Int J Sports Med 1984a; 5:262-267.

Peltenburg AL, Erich WB, Bernink MJ, Zonderland ML, Huisveld IA. Biological maturation, body composition, and growth of female gymnasts and control groups of schoolgirls and girl swimmers, aged 8 to 14 years: A cross-sectional survey of 1064 girls. Int J Sports Med 1984b; 5:36-42.

Roche AF, Chumlea WC Thissen D (1988). Assessing the skeletal maturity of the hand-wrist: Fels Method. Springfield, IL: Charles C Thomas.

Roemmich JN. Weight loss effects on growth, maturation, growth related hormones, protein nutrition markers, and body composition of adolescent wrestlers, Kent State Univ, Dissertation, 1994.

Roemmich JN, Sinning WE. Sport-seasonal changes in body composition, growth, power and strength of adolescent wrestlers. Int J Sports Med 1995, in press.

Roemmich JN, Rogol AD. Physiology of growth and development: Its relationship to performance in the young athlete. Clinics in Sports Medicine 1995; 14:483-502.

Rogol AD, Weltman A, et al. Durability of the reproductive axis in eumenorrheic women during 1 yr of endurance training. J Appl Physiol 1992, 72(4):1571-1580.

Seefeldt V, Haubenstricker J, Branta CF, Evans S. Physical characteristics of adult distance runners. E.W. Brown and C.F. Branta (eds). Competitive Sports for Children and Youth. Champaign, IL: Human Kinetics, 1988, pp. 247-258.

Sidhu LS, Grewal R. Age of menarche in various categories of Indian sports-women. Br J Sports Med 1980; 14:199-203.

Sinning WE, Wilensky N, Meyers E. Post-season body composition changes and weight estimation in high-school wrestlers, in: Broekhoff J. (ed) Physical Education, Sports and the Sciences. Eugene, Oregon, Microform Publications, 1976.

Smith NJ. Weight control in the athlete. Clin Sports Med 1984, 3:693-704.

Steen SN, McKinney S. Nutrition assessment of college wrestlers. Phys Sports Med 1986, 14:100-116.

Steen, SN, Brownell. Patterns of weight loss and regain in wrestlers: Has the tradition changed? Med Sci Sports Exerc 1990, 22, 762-768.

Tanner JM. Foetus into man: Physical growth from conception to maturity. Ware: 1989, Castlemead, 2nd edition.

Tanner JM, Davies PW. Clinical longitudinal standards for height and height velocity for North American children. J Pediatr 1985; 107:317-329.

Tanner JM, Whitehouse RH, Cameron N, Marshall WA, Healy MJR, Goldstein H (1983). Assessment of skeletal maturity and prediction of adult height (2nd ed). New York: Academic Press.

Theintz G, Ladame F, Kehrer E, Plicha C, Howald H, Sizonenko PC. Prospective study of psychological development of adolescent female athletes: Initial assessment. J Adolesc Health 1994a; 15:258-262.

Theintz GE. Endocrine adaption to intensive physical training during growth. Clin Endocrinol 1994b; 41:267-272.

Theintz G, Ladame F, Howald H, Weiss U, Torresani T, Sizonenko PC. The child, growth and high-level sports. Schweizerishche Zeitschrift fur Medizin und Traumatologie, 1994c; 3:7-15.

Theintz GE, Howald H, Weiss U, Sizonenko PC. Evidence for a reduction of growth potential in adolescent female gymnasts. J Peds 1993; 122:306-313.

Tipton, CM, Tcheng TK. Iowa wrestling study. Weight loss in high school wrestlers. JAMA 1970 214, 1269-1274.

Warren MP. The effects of exercise on pubertal progression and reproductive function in girls. J Clin Endocrinol Metab 1980; 51:1150-1157.

Weltman A, Weltman JY, Schurrer R, Evans WS, Veldhuis JD, Rogol AD. Long-term endurance training amplifies the pulsatile release of GH; Effects of training intensity. J Appl Physiol 1992, 72:2188-2196.

Williams MH. Exercise effects on children's health. Gatorade Sport Science Institute. Sports Science Exchange 1993, 4(43).

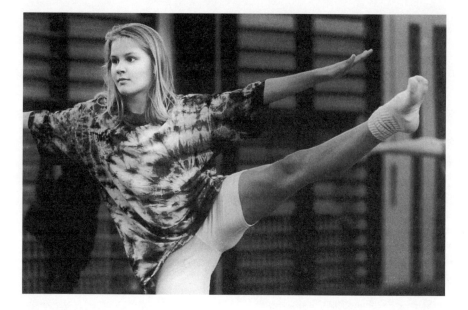

Chapter 5

The Development of Eating Disorders in Young Athletes

Jorunn Sundgot-Borgen and Roald Bahr

Eating disorders (ED) are frequent, and may have long-lasting physical and psychological effects. Symptoms of ED are more prevalent among female athletes than non-athletes (Brownell et al. 1992). Athletes competing in sports where leanness and/or a specific weight are considered important are at increased risk for the development of ED (Brownell et al. 1992 Sundgot-Borgen, 1993a). However, studies show that female athletes competing in sports where weight is considered to be less important, also suffer from ED. Psychological, biological, and social factors inter-relate to produce the clinical picture of ED. New data indicate that specific risk factors for the development of ED occur in sport settings. This article reviews the definition, diagnostic criteria, prevalence and risk factors for the development of ED in sport, as well as practical implications and treatment advice.

Definitions and diagnostic criteria

According to the revised third edition of The Diagnostic and Statistical Manual of Mental Disorders (DSM-III-R);(APA, 1987), ED are characterized by gross disturbances in eating behaviour, and include anorexia nervosa (AN), bulimia nervosa (BN), eating disorder not otherwise specified (EDNOS), pica (craving for unnatural types of food), and rumination disorder (regurgitation of food) in infancy. Binge eating disorder (BED) has only recently been included in the DSM-IV (APA,1994) and has therefore not been examined among athletes. Pica and rumination disorders are generally not a problem in sport. Athletes constitute a unique population and special diagnostic considerations should be made when working with this group (Sundgot-Borgen, 1993a; Szmuckler et al., 1985; Thompson and Sherman, 1993). An attempt has been made to identify the group of athletes who show significant symptoms of ED, but who do not meet the DSM-III-R criteria for AN, BN or NOS (Sundgot-Borgen, 1993a). These athletes have been classified as having a subclinical ED termed anorexia athletica (AA). Health care professionals should be aware of the normal needs, expectations, and performance demands of athletes as this awareness and experience may be helpful in both diagnosis and treatment (Thompson and Sherman, 1993). It is assumed that many cases of AN and BN begin as subclinical variants of these disorders. Early identification and treatment may prevent development of the full disorder (Bassoe, 1990). Finally, subclinical cases are probably more prevalent than those meeting the criteria for AN, BN or BED.

Anorexia nervosa

AN in individuals is characterized by a refusal to maintain body weight over a minimal level considered normal for age and height, a distorted body image, an intense fear of fatness or gaining weight while in fact being underweight and amenorrhea (the absence of at least three consecutive menstrual cycles). Individuals with anorexia "feel fat" while they are in fact underweight (APA, 1987). The diagnostic criteria are listed in table 1.

Table 1: Diagnostic criteria for anorexia nervosa

A. Refusal to maintain body weight over a minimally normal weight for age and height (e.g., weight loss leading to maintenance of body weight 15% below that expected; or failure to make expected weight gain during period of growth, leading to body weight 15% below that expected).
B. Intense fear of gaining weight or becoming fat, even though underweight.
C. Disturbance in the way in which one's body weight or shape is experienced, undue influence of body shape and weight on self-evaluation, or denial of the seriousness of current low body weight.
D. In post-menarcheal females, amenorrhea, i.e., the absence of at least three consecutive menstrual cycles. (A woman is considered to have amenorrhea if her periods occur only following hormone, e.g., estrogen, administration.)

Specify type:
Restricting type: During the episode of Anorexia Nervosa, the person does not regularly engage in binge eating or purging behavior (i.e., self-induced vomiting or the misuse of laxatives or diuretics.)
Binge eating/purging type: During the episode of Anorexia Nervosa, the person regularly engages in binge eating or purging behavior (i.e., self-induced vomiting or the misuse of laxatives or diuretics.)

Bulimia nervosa

Bulimia nervosa is characterized by binge eating (rapid consumption of a large amount of food in a discrete period of time) and purging. This typically involves consumption of high-energy food, usually eaten inconspicuously or secretly. By relieving abdominal discomfort through vomiting, the individual can continue the binge (APA, 1987). The DSM-IV diagnostic criteria for BN include: recurrent episodes of binge eating, inappropriate behaviour to prevent weight gain, the occurence of binge eating and inappropriate compensatory behaviours at least twice a week for at least threee months, and self evaluation based on body shape and weight (APA, 1994) (See table 2).

Table 2: Diagnostic criteria for bulimia nervosa

A. Recurrent episodes of binge eating. An episode of binge eating is characterized by both of the following: (1) eating in a discrete period of time (e.g., within any 2 hour period), an amount of food that is definitely larger than most people would eat during a similar period of time in similar circumstances; and, (2) a sense of lack of control over eating during the episode (e.g., a feeling that one cannot stop eating or control what or how much one is eating).

B. Recurrent inappropriate compensatory behavior in order to prevent weight gain, such as: self-induced vomiting; misuse of laxatives, diuretics or other medications; fasting; or excessive exercise.

C. The binge eating and inappropriate compensatory behaviors both occur, on average, at least twice a week for three months.

D. Self-evaluation is unduly influenced by body shape and weight.

E. The disturbance does not occur exclusively during episodes of Anorexia Nervosa.

Specify type:

Purging type: The person regularly engages in self-induced vomiting or the misuse of laxatives or diuretics.

Non-purging type: The person uses other inappropriate compensatory behaviors, such as fasting or excessive exercise, but does not regularly engage in self-induced vomiting or the misuse of laxatives or diuretics.

Binge eating disorder

BED has recently been added to the DSM-IV criteria (APA, 1994). The primary focus has been on reports of typically overweight patients who binge, but do not purge (Wilson and Walsh, 1991). Indiuviduals with BED have bulimic episodes at least two days a week for six months, but do not meet the criteria for bulimia nervosa (table 3, page 64).

Eating disorder not otherwise specified

The disorders in this category are those that do not meet the criteria for either AN, BN or BED (Wilson and Walsh, 1991). The diagnostic category of EDNOS acknowledges the existence and importance of a variety of eating disturbances

(Thompson and Sherman, 1993). Examples of EDNOS include individuals appearing to have AN, but with regular menses or a normal bodyweight, and individuals who binge eat infrequently (APA, 1994) (Table 4).

Table 3: Diagnostic criteria for binge eating disorder

A. Recurrent episodes of binge eating. An episode of binge eating is characterized by both of the following: (1) eating, in a discrete period of time (e.g., within any 2 hour period), an amount of food that is definitely larger than most people would eat during a similar period of time in similar circumstances; and (2) a sense of lack of control over eating during the episode (e.g., a feeling that one can't stop eating or control what or how much one is eating).

B. The binge eating episodes are associated with at least three of the following:

(1) eating much more rapidly than normal.

(2) eating until feeling uncomfortably full.

(3) eating large amounts of food when not feeling physically hungry.

(4) eating alone because of being embarrassed by how much one is eating.

(5) feeling disgusted with onself, depressed or feeling very guilty after overeating.

C. Marked distress regarding binge eating.

D. The binge eating occurs, on average, at least two days a week* for six months.

E. The disturbance does not occur exclusively during the course of Anorexia Nervosa or Bulimia Nervosa.

*   The method of determining frequency differ from that used for BN; future research should address whether counting the number of days on which binges occur or the number of episodes of binge eating is the preferable method of setting a frequency threshold.

Anorexia athletica

The term AA was first introduced by Pugliese et al. (1983), and the diagnostic criteria have recently been modified (Sundgot-Borgen, 1993) (Table 1). The classic feature of AA is intense fear of gaining weight or becoming fat even though an individual is already lean (at least 5% less than expected normal weight for age and height for the general female population). Weight loss is accomplished by a reduction in energy intake, often combined with extensive or compulsive exercise. The restrictive energy intake is below that required to maintain the energy requirements of the high training volume (Sundgot-Borgen and Larsen, 1993). In addition to normal training to enhance performance in sport, athletes with AA exercise excessively or compulsively to purge their bodies of the effect of eating. These athletes frequently report binge-eating and the use of vomiting, laxatives and/or

Table 4: Diagnostic criteria for eating disorders not otherwise specified, NOS

Disorders of eating that do not meet the criteria for a specific eating disorder. Examples include:

1) all of the criteria for Anorexia Nervosa are met except the individual has regular menses.
2) all of the criteria for Anorexia Nervosa are met except, despite significant weight loss, the individual's current weight is in the normal range.
3) all of the criteria for Bulimia Nervosa are met except binges occur at a frequency of less than twice a week or a duration of less than three months.
4) an individual of normal body weight regularly engages in inappropriate compensatory behavior after eating small amounts of food (e.g., self-induced vomiting after the consumption of two cookies).
5) An individual who repeatedly chews and spits out, but does not swallow, large amounts of food.
6) Binge Eating Disorder: recurrent episodes of binge eating in the absence of inappropriate compensatory behaviors characteristic of bulimia nervosa.

Table 5: Diagnostic criteria for anorexia athletica

1. Weight loss	+
2. Delayed puberty	(+)
3. Menstrual dysfunction	(+)
4. GI complains	(+)
5. Absence of medical illness or affective disorder explaining the weight reduction	+
6. Distorted body image	(+)
7. Excessive fear of becoming obese	+
8. Restriction of food (<1200 kcal/day)	+
9. Use of purging methods	(+)
10. Binge eating	(+)
11. Compulsive exercise	(+)

+: Absolute criteria, (+): relative criteria
1. >5% of expected body weight
2. No menstrual bleeding at age 16 (primary amenorrhea)
3. Primary amenorrhea, secondary amenorrhea and oligomenorrhea
4. Self-induced vomiting, laxatives, and diuretics

diuretics. The binge eating is planned and included in their strict training and study schedule. These athletes often report bingeing. However, their energy intake is usually below the recommended level. Furthermore, it is often difficult for elite athletes to have time for more than two meals to meet energy requirements (Sundgot-Borgen and Larsen, 1993). The term anorexia athletica was first introduced by Pugliese et al. (1983). These criteria were fairly clear and have recently been modified (Table 5) (Sundgot-Borgen, 1993).

Some athletes with AA also meet the criteria of EDNOS. Most athletes have a higher percentage of lean body mass than the average female population, but body-weight more than 5% lower than expected could indicate that an athlete is too lean. Athletes with AA usually indicate that they need to lose weight because of the requierments of their sport or directions from a coach.

Prevalence of eating disorders in athletes

Data on the prevalence of eating disorders in athletic populations is limited and equivocal. Most studies have looked at preoccupation with food, obsessive preoccupation with weight, disturbed body image or the use of pathogenic weight control methods. Almost all investigators who have attempted to study this issue, have used surveys or inventories to establish prevalence of ED, and few have obtained response rates that permit firm conclusions to be drawn. A summary of the studies

Figure 1: Prevalence of eating disorders in female elite athletes representing technical (G1), endurane (G2), aesthetic (G3), weight dependent (G4), ball games (G5) and power sports (G6).

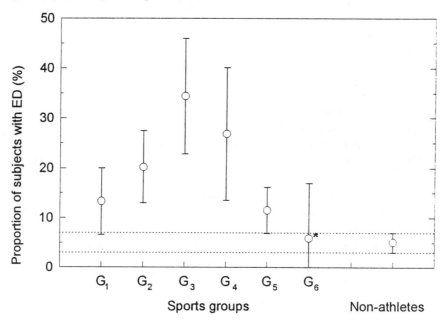

conducted to date have been presented previously (Brownell et al, 1992). Estimates of the prevalence of the symptoms of ED and the existence of ED among athletes range from less than 1% to as high as 39.2% (Warren et al.,1990; Burkes-Miller and Black, 1988). Estimates vary greatly depending on whether they are based on self-reports or clinical interviews and the athletic population investigated. For further methodological discussion see Sundgot-Borgen (1994). Despite methodological weaknesses, studies consistently show that symptoms of ED and pathogenic weight control methods are more frequent in athletes than controls (Smith, 1980; Rosen et al.1986; Sundgot-Borgen and Corbin, 1987, Wilmore, 1991). Also, ED are more prevalent in sports in which leanness and/or a specific weight are considered important.

Elite versus non elite athletes

It is not established whether elite athletes are at greater risk for ED than nonelite athletes. Few studies have specified the competitive level of the athletes investigated. It is assumed that some risk factors (e.g. intense pressure to be lean, increased training volume and perfectionism) are more pronounced in elite athletes. However, it may be assumed that elite athletes would have difficulty performing at an elite level with an ED, since performance would suffer. It is therefore possible that the prevalence of eating disorders and related problems is even higher among athletes who failed to stay at a high performance level. Hamilton et al., (1988) found that less-skilled dancers in the United States reported significantly more eating problems than the more skilled dancers. However, firm conclusions cannot be drawn without longitudinal studies with a careful classification and description of the competitive level of the athletes investigated.

Risk factors for the development of eating disorders

Psychological, biological and social factors are implicated in the development of eating disorders (Garfinkel et al 1987; Katz 1985). Temperament, hunger intensity and activity level contribute to the physiological predisposition. Difficulties in a child's early relationship with the caregiver may create an additional, psychological predisposition (Johnson and Schlundt 1985). Social factors, especially the phenomenon of cultural equating of thinness in women with success, may also contribute (Garner et al.1984). When an individual with a substantial predisposition begins a strict diet, it can become a self-perpetuating, self-reinforcing process (Johnson and Schundt 1985). It has been claimed that female athletes appear to be more vulnerable to eating disorders than the general female population because of additional stresses associated with the athletic environment (Clifton 1991; Wilmore 1991).

The attraction to sport hypothesis

It has been suggested that sport or specific sports attract individuals who are ano-rexic, at least in attitude, if not in behaviour or weight, before commencing their participation in sports (Thompson and Sherman, 1993). These individuals seem to use/abuse exercise to expend extra calories or to justify their abnormal eating and dieting behaviour. Other has suggested that many anorexic individuals are at-tracted to sports in which they can hide their illness (Sacks 1990). The attraction to certain sports such as running and cross-country skiing, may be related to the emphasis on, and acceptance of, thinness and high training volume in those sports. The stereotyped standards of body shape of some sports such as gymnastic and long distance running, make it difficult for observers to notice when a particular athlete has lost too much weight. These common and accepted weight standards help athletes to hide their problem and delay the intervention (Thompson and Sherman 1993). The "attraction to sport" hypothesis appears to have merit in that it covers individuals who already have an ED or are at high risk for developing ED. However, elite gymnasts, for example, are picked to begin intensive, high level training at the age of 6 years, 10 years before developing an eating disorder. Therefore, it would not appear that these individuals were attracted to gymnastics because of a desire for thinness (Thompson and Sherman 1993).

Exercise and the inducement of eating disorders

A bio-behavioral model of activity based AN was proposed in a series of studies by Epling and Piers (1988) and Epling et al.(1983). They suggest that dieting and exercising initiate the anorexic cycle and that as many as 75% of the cases of AN are exercise induced. Specifically, they contend that strenuous exercise tends to suppress appetite, which serves to decrease the value of food reinforcement. As a result, food intake decreases, while the motivation for more exercise increase.

A recent study reported that elite endurance athletes with ED could not give any specific reason why they developed ED (Sundgot-Borgen, 1994). However, many reported that with a sudden increase in training volume, a significant amount of weight was lost and AN or AA developed (Sundgot-Borgen, 1994). Costill (1988) found that athletes who increased their training volume experienced caloric depri-vation. Furthermore, it has been claimed that appetite may be truly diminished, in part as a result of changes in endorphin levels (Katz, 1986). Thus, it has been sug-gested that the increased training load may have induced a caloric deprivation in these endurance athletes which in turn may have elicited biological and social re-inforcements leading to the development of ED (Sundgot-Borgen, 1994). How-ever, not all individuals with AN exercise, and the hypothesis of exercise-induced AN does not explain BN. Thus, longitudinal studies with close monitoring of the training volume, type and intensity of the training in athletes representing different sports are needed before the question regarding the role played by different sport in the development of ED.

Figure 2: General and sport specific factors that can contribute to the development of eating disorders in athletes.

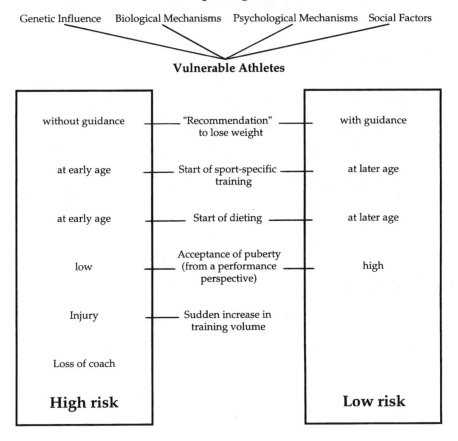

Predisposing factors

Genetic Influence   Biological Mechanisms   Psychological Mechanisms   Social Factors

Vulnerable Athletes

High risk		Low risk
without guidance	"Recommendation" to lose weight	with guidance
at early age	Start of sport-specific training	at later age
at early age	Start of dieting	at later age
low	Acceptance of puberty (from a performance perspective)	high
Injury	Sudden increase in training volume	
Loss of coach		

Early start of sport specific training

It is claimed that an individual's natural body type inherently steers the athlete to an appropriate sport (Brownell et al. 1987). But it is also suggested that the greater the extent to which an athlete's body deviates from the ideal for a particular sport, the greater the risk that the athlete will develop an ED (Brownell et al. 1992). Athletes with ED have been shown to start sport specific training significantly earlier than athletes who do not meet the criteria for ED (Sundgot-Borgen 1994). Starting sport specific training at prepubertal age may have prevented athletes from chosing the sport most suitable for their adult body type.

Hamilton et al. (1988) suggest that dancers who have survived a stringent process of early selection (girls who are enrolled in late childhood and where rigid standards for weight, body shape, and technique must be constantly met) may be more naturally suited to the thin body image demanded by ballet directors, and therefore, less at risk. Furthermore, personal and family history of overweight may be a risk factor for disordered eating because it poses an obstacle to achieving the thinness demanded by some activities such as modern rhythmic gymnastics, gymnastics and long distance running (Garner et al. 1994). The family history should be taken into account when girls chose to compete in a sport at a high level.

Dieting and body weight cycling

Weight cycling usually occurs in athletes who wish to keep weight at a certain level but have difficulty accomplishing this. An example may be a gymnast who wishes to have a low weight to get the best score from the judges. During the off-season weight increases, and restricted eating and/or additional exercise may be necessary to restore the desired weight. Such athletes frequently engage in cycles where they keep their body weight low for periods, but then gain weight due to their restraint weakness or when physiological processes seek to restore a higher body weight (Brownell et al., 1992). In addition to the pressure to reduce weight, athletes are often pressed for time, and they have to lose weight rapidly to make or stay on the team. As a result they often experience frequent periods of restrictive dieting or weight cycling (Sundgot-Borgen, 1994). Periods of restrictive dieting and weight cycling have been suggested as important risk or trigger factors for the development of ED in athletes (Brownell et al., 1987; Sundgot-Borgen,1994). Relatively little information is available on the physiological adaptation of athletes who have restricted their diet and/or have experienced weight cycling over a period of time. The accuracy of self-report and retrospective reports of weight is not known, and there is a need for longitudinal studies (Brownell et al., 1992). However, Steen et al (1988) reported that wrestlers who gain and lose weight repeatedly during training and competition have significantly lower resting metabolic rate (RMR) than nonwrestlers of similar weight, height, and body fat content. It is not known whether the repeated weight gain and losses result in a lower RMR or if there is a subgroup of wrestlers with a low RMR prior to their history of weight cycling (Steen et al., 1988).

Personality factors

The characteristics of a sport (eg. emphasis on leanness or individual competition) may interact with the personality traits of the athlete to start and perpetuate an ED (Wilson and Eldredge, 1992). Some of the personality traits exhibited by athletes in general are similar to traits manifested by many patients with ED. For example, both groups tend to be characterized by high self-expectation, perfectionism, persistence, and independence (Yates, 1991). It may be that these qualities, which enable these individuals to succeed in sports, also place athletes more at risk of developing ED (Yates, 1991). Unfortunately the possible influence that an athlete's personality may have on the development of ED has not been examined. However, experience with athletes with ED lead us to assume that the vulnerability of athletes for ED are compounded by the psychological make up of the elite athlete, who can be described as goal oriented and perfectionistic.

Traumatic events

Some athletes with ED who experienced a significant weight loss without intend-ing to lose weight reported that they had lost their coach or changed coach prior to the weight loss. These athletes all described their coaches as being vital to their fu-ture athletic career (Sundgot-Borgen, 1994). Other athletes reported that they de-veloped ED as a result of an injury or illness that left them temporarily unable to continue their normal level of exercise, as previously described by Katz (1986). Both the loss of coach or unexpected illness or injury can probably be regarded as traumatic events similar to those described as trigger mechanisms for ED in non-athletes (Bassoe, 1990). Sexual abuse by male coaches has also been reported as a possible explanation for the development of ED among some female elite athletes (Sundgot-Borgen,1994).

The impact of coaches and trainers

Pressure to reduce weight has been the general explanation for the increased pre-valence of ED among athletes. A number of investigations report that athletes started dieting after coaches had advised a reduction in weight (Smith, 1980). Many of these athletes are young and extremely impressionable. For them such a recommendation could be seen as a necessary step to achieve success in their sport. However, except from a few studies, the role played by the coaches in this respect has not been examined.

Rosen and Hough (1988) reported that 75% of young athletes who were told by their coaches that they were too heavy, started using pathogenic weight loss meth-ods. However, Rosen and Hough (1988) did not report how many of these young

Table 6: The different reasons for the development of eating disorders re-ported by the eating disorded athletes.

	ED athletes %
Prolonged periods of dieting/weight fluctuations	37
New coach	30
Injury/illness	23
Casual comments	19
Leaving home/failure at school/work	10
Problem in relationship	10
Family problems	7
Illness/injury to family members	7
Death of significant others	4
Sexual abuse	4

Multiple answers were allowed. 15% did not give any specific reason athletes actually developed ED. In our study comparing athletes with ED with those not suffering from ED, results showed that among those who had been told to lose weight but had not developed ED, 75% had received guidance during the weight loss as compared with 10% of those who had developed ED (Sundgot-Borgen, 1994). Therefore, it is not necessarily dieting per se, but whether the athlete receives guidance or not, that is important. The different reasons for the development of ED reported by eating disordered high level athletes are presented in Table 6.

A few studies have examined the educational level among athletes, trainers and athletic trainers (Wolf, 1979; Parr et al. 1984; Sundgot-Borgen, 1993). Findings indicate that too few coaches and trainers in charge of athletes have a formal education in sport or ED (Wolf, 1979, Parr et al.,1984; Sundgot-Borgen, 1993). In Norway, only half of the coaches in charge of the female elite athletes have formal education in physical education and sports. Of those who reportedly supervised athletes during weight loss periods, only coaches with a formal education in sport or physical education followed recommended routines. Furthermore, the coaches in high-prevalence sports (e.g. aesthetic and weight-dependent sports) appeared to have less formally education (Sundgot-Borgen, 1993a) .

The higher prevalence of ED in those groups should not be explained by the low percentages of educated coaches alone, but there may be a connection. For example, the use of pathologic weight control methods such as vomiting, laxatives and diuretics were recommended more frequently by coaches without formal education in physical education. Finally, this study show that coaches with a formal education in physical education have a significantly better knowledge of ED, which is considered important to help them recognize the signs and symptoms of athletes who may have or may develop ED (Sundgot-Borgen, 1993a).

Most researchers agree, however, that coaches do not cause ED in athletes, although trough inappropriate coaching the problem may be triggered or exacerbated in vulnerable individuals (Wilmore, 1991). Therefore, in most cases the role of coaches in the development of ED in athletes should be seen as a part of a complex interplay of factors.

The effects of eating disorders on athletic performance

The psychological and medical features and consequences of ED among athletes and nonathletes have been described and discussed elsewhere (Brownell et al. 1992; Katz 1988; Thompson and Sherman 1993). Laboratory abnormalities and characteristic endocrine abnormalities of ED are discussed by Katz (1988). A number of studies have shown that both athletic controls and athletes suffering from ED who need to keep lean to improve performance, consume surprisingly low amounts of calories (Benson et al 1987; Erp-Bart et al.1985, 1989; Welch et al. 1987). Athletes with ED, except for some of the athletes with BN, consume diets low in energy and key nutrients (Sundgot-Borgen and Larsen 1993). However, the effects of the low energy intake on protein balance have not been studied in detail.

Athletes know that the quickest way to lose weight is by losing body water. Water is essential for the regulating of body temperature, and a dehydrated athlete becomes overheated and fatigued more easily. It has been shown that loss of endurance and coordination due to dehydration can impair exercise performance (Webster et al., 1990). Ingjer and Sundgot-Borgen (1991) reported that elite female endurance athletes with significant reduction of body weight over 2 months showed a significant decrease in maximal oxygen uptake and running speed during the weight reduction period relative to athletes who did not lose weight.

Fasting can also be detrimental to athletic performance. Intense aerobic performance measured as time to exhaustion, declines in cyclists (Loy et al. 1986) and runners after fasting (Nieman et al. 1987). This decline is probably linked to depletion of muscle glycogen, which is less critical for low-intensity than high intensity exercise.

Prevention of eating disorders in athletes

Since the exact causes of ED are unknown, it is difficult to draw up preventive strategies. Coaches should realise that they can strongly influence their athletes. Coaches or other involved with young athletes should not comment on an individual's body size or require weight loss in young and still growing athletes. Without offering further guidance dieting may result in unhealthy eating behaviour or ED in a highly motivated and uninformed athlete (Eisenman et al. 1990). ED are more difficult to treat the longer they progress and, therefore, early intervention is important. However, most important of all is the prevention of circumstances or factors which could lead to an ED. Therefore, professionals working with athletes should be informed about the possible risk factors for the development, early signs and symptoms of ED, the medical, psychological and social consequences of these disorders, how to approach the problem if it occurs and what treatment options are available. This could improve awareness, and facilitate early detection and intervention. While coaches, parents and athletes can learn to identify symptoms that indicate risk, a diagnosis can only be made by a physician or psychologist.

Weight loss recommendation

Some athletes do not have their ideal body composition. Change in body composition and weight loss can be achieved safely if the weight goal is realistic and based on body composition rather than weight-for-height standards. Use of the skinfold appraisal techniques is recommended because of the large time and equipment demands required when using hydrostatic weighing. Following are recommendations for safe weight loss in athletes modified from Eisenman et al.(1990).

Identifying realistic weight goals

Athletes must eat sufficient calories to avoid the loss of muscle tissue, and should start a weight loss program well before the season begins. Changes in body composition should be monitored on a regular basis.

Monitor weight

The coach or others educated in weight-control methods should set realistic goals that address methods of dieting, rate of weight change, and a reasonable target range of weight and body fat. After the athlete has reached the target weight and percentage of body fat, the coach should continue to monitor weight and body composition to detect any continued or unwarranted losses or weight-fluctuation. Private weigh-ins/measurements of body composition to reduce the stress, anxiety, and embarrassment of public assessment should be employed.

Provide nutritional guidance

The coach should not tell athletes to lose weight without providing them with proper nutritional guidance. Rather, the coach should provide a total nutritional program that includes general nutrition counselling as well as help in appropriate methods of weight loss and weight gain. If the coach has no education in nutrition, a registered dietitian, if available, can help individual plan nutritionally adequate diets. Throughout this process, the role of overall, long-term good nutrition practices and weight control in optimizing performance should be emphasized.

Be aware of symptoms

If the athlete exhibit symptoms of an ED, the athlete should be confronted with the possible problem.

Seek professional help

Coaches should not try to diagnose or treat ED, but they should be specific about their suspicions and talk with the athlete about the fears or anxieties they may be having about food and performance. They should support the athlete and reassure them that a team position will not be affected if not medically initiated.

Be a Team Member; The coach should assist and support the athlete during treatment.

Conclusions

There are number of pressing needs for research on athletes and ED. The prevalence of ED is higher among athletes than nonathletes, but the relationship to performance or training level is unknown. Additionally, athletes competing in sports where leanness and/ or a specific weight are considered important are more prone to ED than athletes competing in sports where these factors are considered less important. It appears necessary to examine anorexia nervosa, bulimia nervosa, binge eating disorder, the subclinical disorders and the range of behaviours and attitudes associated with eating disturbances in athletes to learn how these clinical and subclinical disorders are related.

Interesting suggestions about possible sport specific risk factors for the development of ED in athletes exist, but large scale longitudinal studies are needed to learn more about risk factors and the etiology of ED in athletes at different competitive levels and within different sports.

More knowledge about the short and long term effects of ED upon the health and performance of athletes is needed.

References

American Psychiatric Association. Diagnostic and Statistical Manual of Mental Disorders, Third Edition-Revised (DSM-III-R), p, 65-69. Washington, DC, 1987.

American Psychiatric Association. Diagnostic and Statistical Manual of Mental Disorders, pp. 1-2, 4th ed. (DSM-IV), American Psychiatric Association DC, 1994.

Bassoe HH. Anorexia/Bulimia Nervosa: The development of anorexia nervosa and of mental symptoms. Treatment and the outcome of the disease. Acta Psychiatrica Scandinavia 82 (suppl.) 7-13, 1990.

Benson J, Gillien DM, Bourdet K, Loosli AR. Inadequate nutrition and chronic calorie restriction in adolescent ballerinas. Physician and Sportsmedicine 13:79-90, 1985.

Brownell KD, Rodin J, Wilmore JH. Eating, body weight and performance in athletes. Disorders of modern society (Eds), Philadelphia; Lea and Febiger, 1992.

Brownell KD, Steen SN, Wilmore JH. Weight regulation practices in athletes: Analysis of metabolic and health effects. Medicine and Science in Sports and Exercise 6:546-556, 1987.

Burckes-Miller ME, Black DR. Male and female college athletes. Prevalence of anorexia nervosa and bulimia nervosa. Athletic Training 2:137-140, 1988.

Clifton EJ. Eating disorders in female athletes: Identification and management. Kentuckey AHPERD Journal (27) 1:30-32, 1991.

Costill DL. Carbohydrate for exercise: Dietary demands for optimal performance. International Journal of Sportsmedicine 9:1-18, 1988.

Davis C, Cowls MA. A comparison of weight and dieting concerns and personality factors among female athletes and non-athletes. Journal of Psychosomatic Research 33:527-536, 1989.

Dummer GM, Rosen LW, Heusner WW et al. Pathogenic weight-control behaviors of young competitive swimmers. Physician and Sportsmedicine 5:75-86, 1987.

Eisenman PA, Johnson SC, Benson JE. Coaches guide to nutrition and weight control (second edition) p 129-140. Leisure Press Champaign, Illinois, 1990.

Epling WF, Pierce WD, Stefan L. A theory of activitybased anorexia. International Journal of Eating Disorders 3:27-46, 1983.

Epling WF, Pierce WD. Activity based anorexia nervosa. International Journal of Eating Disorders 7:475-485, 1988.

Erp-Bart AM, Saris RA, Binkhorst JA, Elvers JWH. Nationwide survey on nutrient habits in elite athletes. Energy, carbohydrates, protein and fat intake. International Journal of Sportsmedicine 10:3-10, 1989.

Erp-Bart AMJ, Fredrix LWHM, Binkhorst RA et al. Energyintake and energy expenditure in top female gymnasts, in Brinkhorst et al (Eds): Children and Exercise XI. Champaign, IL. University Park Press p 218-223, 1985.

Garfinkel PE, Garner DM, Goldbloom DS. Eating disorders implications for the 1990's. Canadian Journal of Psychiatry 32:624-631, 1987.

Garner DM, Garfinkel PE. An index of symptoms of anorexia nervosa. Psychological Medicine 9:273-279, 1979.

Garner DM, Olmsted MP. Polivy J. Manual of Eating Disorder Inventory (EDI). Odessa: Psychological Assessment Resourches, 1984.

Hamilton LH, Brocks-Gunn J, Warren MP. Sociocultural influences on eating disorders in professional female ballet dancers. International Journal of Eating Disorders 4:465-477, 1985.

Hamilton LH, Brooks-Gunn J, Warren MP, Hamilton WG. The role of selectivity in the pathogenesis of eating problems in ballet dancers. Medicine and Science in Sports And Exercise 20:560-565, 1988.

Ingjer F, Sundgot-Borgen J. Influence of body weight reduction on maximal oxygen uptake in female elite athletes. Scandinavian Journal of Medicine and Science in Sports 1:141-146, 1991.

Johnson WG, Schlundt DG. Eating disorders: Assessment and treatment. Clinical Obstetritics and Gynecology 3:598-614, 1985.

Katz JL. Some reflections on the nature of the eating disorders. International Journal of Eating Disorders 4, 617-626, 1985.

Katz JL. Long-distance running, anorexia nervosa, and bulimia: A report of two cases. Comprehensive Psychiatry 1:74-78, 1986.

Katz JL. Eating disorders in women and exercise. In Shangold and Mirken (Eds) Physiology and Sports Medicine p 248-263, F.A. Davis Company. Philadelphia, 1988.

Loy SF. et al. Effects of 24-hour fast on cycling endurance time at two different intensities. Journal of Applied Physiology 61:654-, 1986.

Mallick MJ, Whipple TW, Huerta E. Behavioral and psychological traits of weight-conscious teenagers: A comparison of eating disordered patients and high-and low risk groups. Adolescence 22:157-167, 1987.

Meredith CN, Stern JS. Nutrient intake and the regulation of body weight and body composition. In Brownell et al (Eds) Eating, body weight and performance in athletes. Disorders of Modern Society p 45-60, Philadelphia: Lea and Feibiger, 1992.

Nieman C et al. Running endurance in 27-h fasted humans. Journal of Applied Physiology 63:2503, 1987.

Parr RB, Porter MA, Hodgson SC. Nutrient knowledge and practice of coaches, trainers, and athletes. Physician and Sportsmedicine 3:127-138, 1984.

Rosen LW, Hough DO. Pathogenic weight-control behaviors of female college gymnasts. Physician and Sportsmedicine 9:141-144, 1988.

Rosen LW, McKeag DB, Hough DO et al. Pathogenic weight-control behaviors in female athletes. Physician and Sportsmedicine 14:79-86, 1986.

Sacks MH. Psychiatry and sports. Annals of Sports Medicine 5:47-52, 1990.

Smith NJ. Excessive weight loss and food aversion in athletes simulating anorexia nervosa Pediatrics 66 (1):139-143, 1980.

Steen SN, Brownell KD. Current patterns of weight loss and regain in wrestlers: Has the tradition changed? Medicine and Science in Sports and Exercise 22:762-768, 1990.

Steen SN, Oppliger RA, Brownell KD. Metabolic effects of repeated weight loss and regain in adolescent wrestlers. Journal of the American Medical Associations 260:47-50, 1988.

Sundgot-Borgen J. Prevalence of eating disorders in female elite athletes. International Journal of Sports Nutrition 3:29-40, 1993.

Sundgot-Borgen J. Risk and trigger factors for the development of eating disorders in female elite athletes. Medicine and Science in Sports and Exercise. vol. 26, No. 4, pp. 414-419, 1994.

Sundgot-Borgen J, Larsen S. Nutrient intake and eating behavior of female elite athletes suffering from anorexia nervosa, anorexia athletica and bulimia nervosa. International Journal of Sport Nutrition 3:431-442, 1993.

Sundgot-Borgen J, Brownell KD. Prevalence of eating disorders in male and female athletes, submitted.

Sundgot Borgen J, Corbin CB. Eating disorders among female athletes. Physician and Sportsmedicine 2:89-95, 1987.

Szmuckler GI, Eisler I, Gillis I et al. The implications of anorexia nervosa in a ballet school. Journal of Psychiatric Research 19:177-181, 1985.

Warren BJ, Stanton AL, Blessing DL. Disorded eating patterns in competitive female athletes. International Journal of Eating Disorders 5:565-569, 1990.

Welch PK, Zager KA, Endres J et al. Nutrition Education, body composition and dietary intake of female college athletes. The Psysician and Sportsmedicine 15:63-74, 1987.

Webster S, Rutt R, Weltman A. Physiological effects of weight loss regimen practiced by college wrestlers. Medicine and Science in Sports and Exercise 22:229-233, 1990.

Wilmore JH. Eating and weight disorders in female athletes. International Journal of Sport Nutrition 1:104-117, 1991.

Wilson T, Eldredge KL. Pathology and development of eating disorders: Implications for athletes. In Brownell et al., (Eds) Eating, body weight and performance in athletes. Disorders of Modern Society, Philadelphia: Lea and Febiger, 1992.

Wilson GT, Walsh BT. Eating disorders in the DSM-IV. Journal of Abnormal Psychology 3:362-365, 1991.

Wolf EMB, Wirth JC, Lohman TG. Nutritional practices of coaches in the Big Ten. Physician and Sports Medicine 2:112-124, 1975.

Yates A. Compulsive exercise and eating disorders. New York: Brunner/Mazel, 1991.

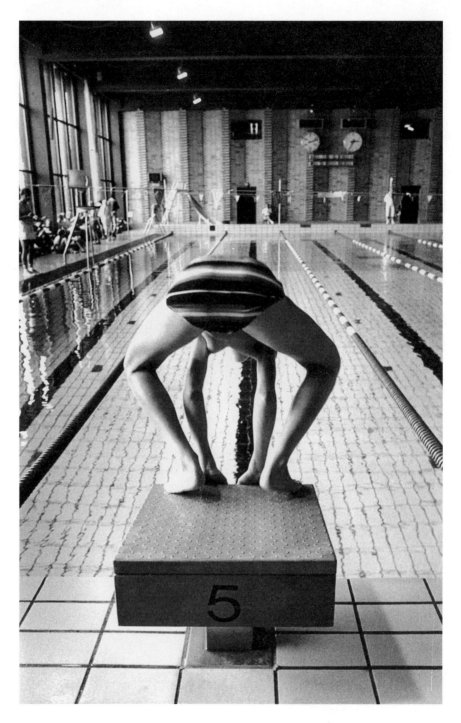

Chapter 6

Tracking in Body Composition and Risk Factors for Cardiovascular Disease from Childhood to Middle Age

Alex F. Roche

Abstract

The analysis of tracking should be an integral part of most longitudinal studies. It is particularly important for studies that include variables with clear relationships to health and for studies that extend to ages when diseases that can be linked to childhood status become common. Analyses of tracking from the Fels Longitudinal Study are used as examples of a larger literature. Age-to-age correlations, which are considered first, may be between values at two ages, or between the means of values during a younger age range and status values at an older age, or between the coefficients of a model fitted to serial data for a younger age range and either corresponding coefficients or status values at older ages. Other approaches include the fitting of parametric or non-parametric mathematical models, the estimation of the extent of canalization, and the calculation of the risk of values in adulthood that are associated with increased probability of disease dependent upon the values of single or multiple variables during childhood.

Introduction

Analyses of data collected in longitudinal growth studies have become more interesting and more complex in recent years. These changes have occurred because of improved computer techniques and the development of new statistical procedures. Despite these advances, the analysis of tracking is difficult particularly if it involves the management of a large complex data base for a study that is still in progress. Due to space limitations, this account will be restricted to findings from the Fels Longitudinal Study. The nature of this study, and an outline of the findings from it, are given in Roche (1992). Other important reports are noted and discussed in the references listed with this paper. Many tracking analyses relate to the calculation of increments between examinations separated by intervals of one year or less, but these are of limited value. Some relate to changes and continuities during longer time intervals; a few use data that extend from childhood to middle age. These unusual data, many of which were collected without a clear vision of their utility, provide opportunities to address topics of great interest.

A popular American dictionary defines tracking as "the maintenance of a constant distance between a pair of wheels traveling in a straight line". This is shown diagramatically in Figure 1a. Modifying this over-specific concept, a biological variable is said to track if, during a period of time, the differences between pairs of individuals for the values of a variable remain constant or, the rank order of the values among a set of individuals is maintained (Figure 1b). These and related phenomena can be analyzed in various ways to provide findings that are usually applicable to groups but may be applicable to individuals.

Figure 1: A diagrammatic representation of tracking. 1a – the dictionary concept; 1b – exact tracking for variables that increase with time; 1c – changes with time that would indicate exact tracking if correlations are calculated between the sets of first and last values but not if data at intermediate ages are considered.

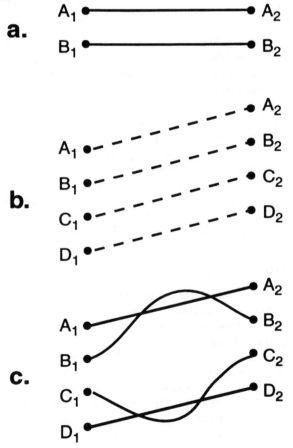

Correlations between repeated measures

In their simplest form, correlations between repeated measures are calculated from values for one variable measured in a group of individuals at two ages. The correlation coefficients summarize the extent to which the differences between individuals, or the rank order of values, are retained from one age to another. This is the method of choice for the analysis of tracking in continuous variables when data are available at only two ages in each individual, but they provide incomplete information about tracking. For example, correlations between the set of data at entry and the set at exit from the study, shown diagrammatically in Figure 1b, would indicate complete tracking. If each individual were measured at numerous ages, a matrix of age-to-age correlations based on pairs of values could be calculated. This might show incomplete tracking to intermediate ages (Figure 1c). In such correlations, the earlier value can be the mean of measurements at several ages or a coefficient of a mathematical model fitted to the serial data for a set of younger ages. Similar considerations apply to the value for the older age.

Age-to-age correlations are commonly influenced by the age at the first measurements, the length of the intervals between measurements, the variability of the changes in the measure during the interval, and the precision of the measurements. Furthermore, and this applies to most studies of tracking, the extent to which the results can be generalized is limited because the data rarely, if ever, come from random samples and, if some of the data were collected a long time ago, there may

Figure 2: Correlations between values for body mass index (BMI) in childhood with those at 35 yrs (Guo et al., 1994. Reproduced with permission from the American Journal of Clinical Nutrition)

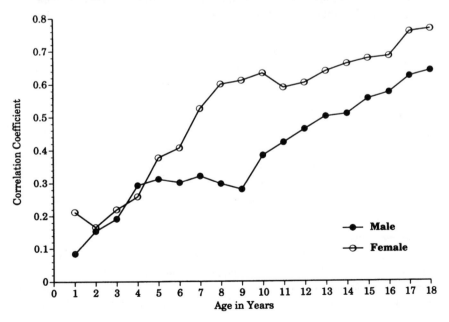

have been marked changes in those environmental conditions that can affect growth.

Weight and body mass index

There are low correlations between weight at 30 years and weights at birth and one year (r = 0.1 to 0.4). These correlations increase to be about 0.7 in girls and 0.5 in boys for childhood values recorded at 8 years, but there are only slow increases in the correlations as older childhood ages are considered. A major feature is that the correlations are higher for girls than boys .

Figure 2 shows a similar pattern of correlations for weight/stature^2 (BMI) in childhood with values at 35 years (Guo et al., 1994). Thus there is greater tracking from childhood to adulthood in weight and in BMI for females than for males after 6 years. For weight and for BMI, the low correlations between values in infancy and those in adulthood lead to the conclusion that there is only a slight tendency for overweight infants to become overweight adults.

Similar conclusions were reached by Kouchi et al., 1985a) who fitted a model to serial weight data for infancy and correlated the coefficients of this model with weight at 18 years and at 30 years. These correlations are significant for the coefficients of θ_1 (intercept) and of θ_2 (linear slope) with values at 18 years and for the coefficients of θ_2 with values at 30 years, but only one of the correlations including the non-linear slope parameter (θ_3) is significant (Table 1). These findings indicate limited but real tracking of weight from birth to 18 years and to 30 years, that is influenced by size at birth and the linear changes during infancy.

Table 1: Correlations between the coefficients of models fitted to serial data during infancy and status at 18 and 30 years (data from Kouchi et al., 1985a,b)

		Males			Females		
		$\hat{\theta}_1$	$\hat{\theta}_2$	$\hat{\theta}_3$	$\hat{\theta}_1$	$\hat{\theta}_2$	$\hat{\theta}_3$
Weight	18 yrs	.21*	.25**	.21*	.23**	.26**	–
	30 yrs	–	.23*	–	–	.39**	–
Recumbent length/stature	18 yrs	.33**	.45**	–	.36**	.35**	–

The coefficients are those of the model: $y_{ij} = \theta_{1i} + \theta_{2i} + t_{ij}{}^\theta 3i + \epsilon_{ij}$
Only significant correlations are shown.

Recumbent length and stature

Almost *a priori*, one would expect more tracking in recumbent length and stature than in weight since the changes in recumbent length and stature across age are more regular and are monotonic. Age-to-age correlations between childhood statures and stature at 18 years are high even for long intervals (Table 2). The correla-

Table 2: Correlations between stature in childhood and at 18 years

Childhood age (yrs)	Males	Females
4	.82	.69
6	.81	.72
8	.82	.73
10	.82	.63
12	.74	.74
16	.93	.99

tions with values at 12 years in boys and 10 years in girls tend to be low compared with the general trend which suggests tracking of stature is reduced early in pubescence.

Kouchi et al. (1985b) fitted the same model to recumbent length during infancy that they had previously fitted to weight. Selected correlations between the coefficients of the model and stature at 18 years are given in Table 1. In each sex, the correlations with values at 18 years are significant for θ_1 and θ_2 but not for θ_3 indicating that recumbent length during infancy tracks to adult stature. This tracking is influenced by the initial level and the linear rate of change during infancy but not by the non-linear rate of change. The correlation coefficients are larger than those for weight but are only moderate (0.33 to 0.45).

Correlations have been reported between coefficients of longitudinal principal component models fitted to serial data for BMI during 3- to 7-year periods at ages during childhood and adolescence (Cronk et al., 1982a). The first component describes the general level of the recorded values. The correlations for the coefficients of this component for birth to 3 years with those for 3 to 9 years are about 0.6, and the correlations for the period from birth to 3 years with those for 10 to 17 years are about 0.4. The correlations for the coefficients for the first component from 3 to 9 years with those for 10 to 17 years are about 0.8. The age-to-age correlations for the coefficients of the second component, which reflects the rate of change, are low ($r \approx 0.2$) between all pairs of age periods. These findings suggest that the mean levels of BMI during selected age ranges show modest tracking from infancy to childhood but little tracking from infancy to adolescence. There is, however, considerable tracking from childhood to adolescence which is influenced only slightly by the rate of change in BMI during these age ranges.

The same model was used to analyze relationships between BMI during childhood and selected measures of body fatness in adulthood (Cronk et al., 1982b). Multiple regressions show the childhood coefficients for BMI explain about 50% of the variance in BMI at 30 years. The significant coefficients with percent body fat at 30 years are those for component 1 at 4-18 years in males and those for components 1 at birth-3 years and 10-17 years in females. The R^2 values are 0.3 for males and 0.4 for females.

Adipose tissue thicknesses

Age-to-age correlations for subcutaneous adipose tissue thicknesses at many sites have been reported from the major US longitudinal growth studies (Roche, et al., 1982). The correlations between values at 16 years and those at younger ages are higher for females than for males until 6 years after which they are about 0.6 in each sex. Age-to-age correlations between ratios of skinfold thicknesses, which are indices of adipose tissue distribution, at 14 years with those at younger ages are about 0.4 (Baumgartner & Roche, 1988). In males but not females, the correlations for these ratios are lower when the intervals between measurements are longer.

Lipids and lipoproteins

A linear model that allowed for unequal time intervals between measurements and for missing data was used to analyze tracking of plasma lipids and lipoproteins from 9 to 21 years (Guo et al., 1993). With this approach, all the data were included in one analysis that allowed the tracking coefficients to vary with the lengths of the intervals between the measurements. For intervals of 2 to 10 years, the coefficients tend to be higher (r = 0.4 to 0.7) for total cholesterol and LDL-cholesterol than for HDL-cholesterol (r = 0.1 to 0.5). The coefficients decrease slightly as longer intervals are considered.

Blood pressures

Age-to-age correlations from a damped autoregressive model have been reported for blood pressures (Beckett et al., 1992). Of particular interest in the present context are those between values at 13 to 16 years and those recorded 4 to 28 years

---

Table 3: Blood pressure pairwise correlations in the Fels Longitudinal Study

Sex and age (years) at first measurements	4	8	Interval (yrs) 16	20	24	28
			Systolic			
Males, 13-16	0.39	0.19	0.24	0.21	0.30	0.43
	(213)	(141)	(94)	(65)	(57)	(45)
Females, 13-16	0.42	0.44	0.16	0.14	0.23	0.25
	(206)	(129)	(84)	(69)	(47)	(46)
			Diastolic			
Males, 13-16	0.40	0.16	0.08	0.32	0.17	0.05
	(206)	(130)	(87)	(60)	(51)	(39)
Females, 13-16	0.34	0.16	0.28	0.17	0.29	0.06
	(199)	(125)	(81)	(66)	(42)	(42)

N in parentheses

later at about 17 to 44 years of age (Table 3). The coefficients are generally low (r = 0.1 to 0.4), but they tend to be higher than those reported by others. This may be due to the use of mean values when there were multiple examinations during an age range. The coefficients differ little between males and females or between systolic and diastolic pressures. They tend to decrease slightly as longer intervals between measurements are considered, but they are not closely related to the age at the first measurement.

In summary, age-to-age correlations show considerable age-related and sex-related differences in the tracking of weight and BMI, marked tracking for stature, modest tracking for adipose tissue thicknesses, and little tracking for ratios of these thicknesses. Furthermore, there are differences in the extent of tracking for various lipids and lipoproteins and only a limited tracking of blood pressures. These findings are relevant to some public health issues and could be useful in research planning, but they are not applicable to individuals.

Fit of parametric models

Parametric mathematical models can summarize serial data for individuals by defining the shapes of the growth curves for individuals, the differences in these curves among individuals, and how closely individuals follow their own predicted curves. They can also be used to estimate points on the curves of biological interest, e.g., ages at peak height velocity. Such models can help to evaluate tracking from childhood to adulthood, to predict adulthood values from childhood values, and to estimate the effects of independent variables.

If a parametric model fits well to serial data for individuals, it can be concluded that the individuals have similar growth patterns although these patterns may differ in levels and in the timing of inflections or other changes. It is necessary to choose a parametric model that fits well. Guo et al. (1992) showed that the double logistic and the Preece-Baines models fit poorly to serial data for stature (Bock et al., 1973; Preece & Baines, 1978), but the triple logistic model of Bock and Thissen (1980) fits well. This implies there is considerable tracking of stature which is shown also by high age-to-age correlations (Table 2).

The poor fit of the Preece-Baines model is important not only in relation to tracking but because this model is used commonly to derive biological parameters from serial stature data. The Preece-Baines estimates differ markedly from estimates made from the triple logistic model or from a non-parametric method, kernel regression, which also fits very well. The Preece-Baines model does not describe the mid-growth spurt, it estimates ages at peak height velocity that are 6 months too young, and it provides a rate of growth at peak height velocity that is 1.4 cm x year^{-1} too slow (Guo et al., 1992).

Fit of non-parametric models

A 4-parameter polynomial model was fitted to logarithmic-transformed serial data for BMI (Siervogel et al., 1991). The model fitted well and provided estimates of some biological parameters that were significantly correlated with BMI at 18 years. These biological parameters were: Minimum value (r = 0.5), age at minimum value (r = − 0.5), and maximum velocity (r = 0.8). The corresponding correlation with the age at maximum velocity was not significant. These findings provide important information about tracking. If applied to the type of data shown in Figure 1c, they would indicate that tracking is far from complete because one model would not fit all individuals.

Canalization

The zone between adjacent percentile lines on a growth chart can be called a canal. For example, this zone or canal may be bounded by the 10th and 25th percentile lines. If serial data points for an individual stay in the same canal, the child's growth is said to be canalized. Pediatricians commonly identify changes in the growth patterns of children by noting whether their serial data points cross two percentile lines. When this occurs, the growth curve for the child has moved from one zone, across another, to a third. Little is known of the prevalence of such changes. Smith et al. (1976), who analyzed data from a small sample, reported that a failure of canalization occurred for length in 23% of infants between birth and

Figure 3: The 75th, 85th and 95th percentiles for body mass index (BMI; kg x m⁻²) in males from the second National Health and Nutrition Examination Survey (US). Segments of the percentile lines are differentially shaded to indicate differences in the probability that BMI at 35 yrs will be > 28 kg x m⁻². (Guo et al., 1994. Reproduced with permission from the American Journal of Clinical Nutrition)

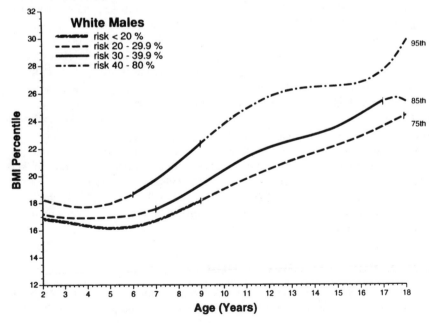

two years. Berkey et al. (1983), who analyzed data from birth to six years, calculated the probabilities of all possible changes. Their results are symmetrical because the analyses were made of the total data base. Had sub-groups of their sample, for example, children with lower initial percentile levels, been analyzed separately, the results may have differed. Better analyses are required that take account of the initial level, the length of the interval, and covariates including the maturity of the child and parental size. The results of such analyses would be specific to the reference data chosen, but they would be valuable for application to individuals in clinical circumstances.

The patterns of change illustrated in Figure 1c can be analyzed using Foulkes-Davis indices (1981) which provide information that is conceptually relevant to canalization. These indices are derived from the number of crossings by curves that were next in rank order at the beginning of the age interval, in relation to the maximum possible number of such crossings. This is a research approach since it requires many serial data points for each individual. Canalization, however, is usually evaluated by clinicians when there are few serial data points for each patient.

Figure 4: The 75th, 85th and 95th percentiles for body mass index (BMI; kg x m^{-2}) in females from the second National Health and Nutrition Examination Survey (US). Segments of the 75th, 85th, and 95 percentile lines are differentially shaded to indicate differences in the probability that BMI at 35 yrs will be > 26 kg x m^{-2}. (Guo et al., 1994. Reproduced with permission from the American Journal of Clinical Nutrition)

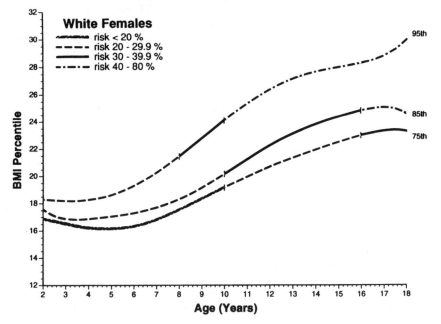

Univariate risk analysis

Guo et al. (1994) analyzed the relationships between annual BMI values during childhood and BMI values larger than the recommended upper limits at 35 years (males > 28 kg x m^{-2}; females > 26 kg x m^{-2}). The probabilities (risks) of high values in adulthood were calculated in relation to BMI reference percentiles from the second National Health and Nutrition Examination Survey (US; 1976-1980) that were published by Najjar and Rowland (1987). The findings were plotted in formats that can assist the clinical management of overweight children (Figures 3 and 4). It is suggested that a clinician who recognizes that a child is overweight should calculate BMI and plot the value on Figure 3 or 4 depending on the sex of the child. The shading of these percentile lines should be noted. A boy aged 10 years at the 85th percentile level for BMI can be told he is a member of a group of boys with a probability of 30-39.9% that the value for BMI at 35 years will be larger than the recommended upper limit. Admittedly, about 60-70% of this group will not have a larger than recommended value of BMI at 35 years. Nevertheless, there should be concern about the increased risk of a large BMI value in adulthood and the expectation that the mean life span for the group to which the boy belongs will be reduced due to an increased prevalence of some diseases such as diabetes mellitus.

Other analyses have shown that the risk of diastolic pressure > 90 mmHg at 35 years is greatly increased for children with high diastolic pressures (Beckett al., 1992). These risks were calculated relative to those of children whose diastolic pressures were 60 mmHg which is near the median value. For example, the relative risks of high diastolic pressures at 35 years are 1.9 for boys and 2.6 for girls who have with diastolic pressures of 80 mmHg at 15 years. Additionally, Guo et al. (1993) reported risk analyses of lipids and lipoproteins from 9 to 21 years. As an example, using a nationally recommended upper limit of 3.36 mmol x l^{-1} for LDL-cholesterol, the risk that the value at 21 years will be larger than the recommended upper limit is 2.7 for a boy or girl with a value of 2.97 mmol x l^{-1} at 9 to 11 years, relative to the risk for a child with a value of 2.46 mmol x l^{-1} at that age.

Multivariate risk analysis

It is probable that the confidence limits of the risks estimated from univariate analyses would be reduced if other variables were considered. Multivariate risk analyses are planned of (i) adult blood pressure dependent on childhood blood pressure and body mass index and parental blood pressure, (ii) adult BMI dependent on childhood and parental BMI, and (iii) adult lipids and lipoproteins dependent on the corresponding childhood values, childhood BMI and parental values for lipids, lipoproteins and BMI.

The significance of tracking

Longitudinal studies of child growth have been conducted in many countries at great expense and with the support of dedicated teams of scientists. These studies have provided many sets of normative data that can be applied by clinicians and epidemiologists. More such studies are needed particularly where there are rapid environmental changes and they are needed of children with pathological conditions. Such growth studies should not be limited to anthropometry and the estimation of maturity. They should, to the extent that resources allow, include measures of body composition and of risk factors for disease, and should record data for factors, such as specific genes, that can influence these measures. The relationships between childhood variables and risk factors for adult disease should be studied since the findings could assist clinical intervention for individuals and the design of public health programs.

A common question is: When does growth stop? Of course, growth does not stop. Mucosal cells divide throughout life and various other changes continue, some of which could be labelled "negative growth." Therefore, it is clear that, in the ideal world, growth studies would continue throughout the life span. There are still some, however, who believe a human growth study should stop at 18 years. Why?

References

Baumgartner RN, Roche AF: Tracking of fat pattern indices in childhood: The Melbourne Growth Study. Hum. Biol. 60:549-567, 1988.

Beckett LA, Rosner B, Roche AF, Guo S: Serial changes in blood pressure from adolescence into adulthood. Am. J. Epid. 10:1166-1177, 1992.

Berkey CS, Reed RB, Valadian I: Longitudinal growth standards for preschool children. Ann. Hum. Biol. 10:57-67, 1983.

Bock RD, Thissen D: Statistical problems of fitting individual growth curves, In: Human Physical Growth and Maturation: Methodologies and Factors, F. E. Johnston, A. F. Roche, and C. Susanne (eds): New York, Plenum. pp 265-290, 1980.

Bock RD, Wainer H, Petersen A, Thissen D, Murray J, Roche AF: A parameterization for individual human growth curves. Hum. Biol. 45:63-80, 1973.

Cronk CE, Roche AF, Kent R, Berkey C, Reed RB, Valadian I, Eichorn D, McCammon R: Longitudinal trends and continuity in weight/stature^2 from 3 months to 18 years. Hum. Biol. 54:729-749, 1982a.

Cronk CE, Roche AF, Chumlea WC, Kent R: Longitudinal trends of weight/stature^2 in childhood in relationship to adulthood body fat measures. Hum. Biol. 54:751-764, 1982b.

Foulkes MA, Davis CE: An index of tracking for longitudinal data. Biometrics 37:439-446, 1981.

Guo S, Beckett L, Chumlea WC, Roche AF, Siervogel RM: Serial analysis of plasma lipid and lipoproteins from 9 to 21 years. Am. J. Clin. Nutr. 58:61-67, 1993.

Guo SS, Roche AF, Chumlea WC, Gardner JD, Siervogel RM: The predictive value of childhood body mass index values for overweight at age 35 y. Am. J. Clin. Nutr. 59:810-819, 1994.

Guo S, Siervogel RM, Roche AF, Chumlea Wm C: Mathematical modelling of human growth: A comparative study. Am. J. Hum. Biol. 4:93-104, 1992.

Kouchi M, Mukherjee D, Roche AF: Curve fitting for growth in weight during infancy with relationships to adult status, and familial associations of the estimated parameters. Hum. Biol. 57:245-265, 1985a.

Kouchi M, Roche AF, Mukherjee D: Growth in recumbent length during infancy with relationships to adult status and familial associations of the estimated parameters. Hum. Biol. 57:449-472, 1985b.

Najjar MF, Rowland M: Anthropometric Reference Data and Prevalence of Overweight. United States, 1976-80. Vital and Health Statistics, Series 11, No. 238, National Center for Health Statistics 1-73, 1987.

Preece MA, Baines MJ: A new family of mathematical models describing the human growth curve. Ann. Hum. Biol. 5:1-24, 1978.

Roche AF: Growth, Maturation and Body Composition: The Fels Longitudinal Study 1929-1991. Cambridge, United Kingdom, Cambridge University Press, 1992.

Roche AF, Siervogel RM, Chumlea WC, Reed RB, Valadian I, Eichorn D, McCammon RW: Serial Changes in Subcutaneous Fat Thicknesses of Children and Adults. Monographs in Paediatrics, Vol. 17. Basel, Karger, 1982.

Siervogel RM, Roche AF, Guo S, Mukherjee D, Chumlea WC: Patterns of change in weight/stature^2 from 2 to 18 years: Findings from long-term serial data for children in the Fels Longitudinal Growth Study. Int. J. Obesity 15:478-485, 1991.

Smith DW, Troug W, Rogers JE, Greitzer LJ, Skinner AL, McCann JJ, Harvey MAS: Shifting linear growth during infancy: Illustration of genetic factors in growth from fetal life through infancy. Pediatrics 89:225-230, 1976.

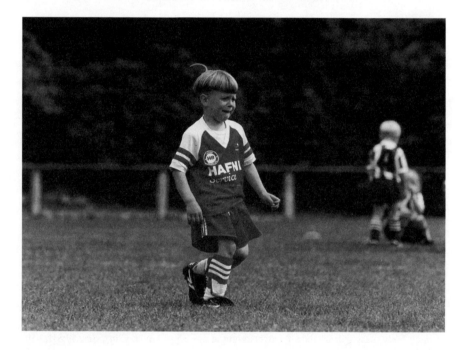

Chapter 7

Early Primary Hypertension in Children and Implications for Prevention: The Role of Physical Fitness.

Henrik S. Hansen

Blood pressure elevation in adulthood is a well established risk factor for cardio-vascular morbidity and mortality. Increasing evidence suggests a causal association and that the roots of essential hypertension extend back into childhood (Lever and Harrap 1992) and intrauterine growth (Barker et al 1993).

So far, no blood pressure data are available from groups of individuals followed from infancy into adulthood, and the predictive value of blood pressure in child-hood for hypertensive disease in adulthood is unknown. Several sources of evidence, however, suggest a tendency for blood pressure to retain its rank or position over time, a phenomenon called »tracking«. The view that primary hypertension may have its genesis in childhood has evoked many studies of level, course and determinants of blood pressure in childhood. Of particular interest are the questions concerning which levels of blood pressure are »normal« or, conversely »abnormal«, and reference values for blood pressure in North-American (Task Force Working Group 1987) and European children (de Man et al 1991) have been published. Understanding this phenomenon is important because early prevention would interrupt the natural course of essential hypertension and reduce cardiovascular morbidity and mortality.

In adults, physical training has been followed by a coincident blood pressure reduction in hypertensives and in normal subjects, and an independent preventive effect of a high level of sustained physical activity on coronary heart disease mortality has been demonstrated. Thus physical training might prove an important non-pharmacological approach to primary prevention of essential hypertension.

This paper focuses on (1) some of the evidence that essential hypertension begins in early life, (2) the relationship between physical fitness and blood pressure in children, and (3) prospective training studies in children for controlling blood pressure.

Evidence that essential hypertension begins in early life

Autopsy studies of young individuals dying accidentally and who previously participated in the Bogalusa Heart Study, indicate small renal artery changes and atherosclerotic lesions in the aorta and coronary vessels, and an association between these changes with higher blood pressure levels (Berenson et al 1994). These results are in accordance with the concept that hypertension plays a role in acceleration of atherosclerosis.

Echocardiographic studies have demonstrated that increased left ventricular mass is a strong predictor of cardiovascular morbidity in hypertensive adults (Devereux 1989), and appears to be a risk factor independent of blood pressure, for subsequent coronary heart disease events (Koren et al 1991).

Comparative studies of children in the upper 5-10 percentile of the blood pressure distribution with those form the lower part have demonstrated significant increases in both left ventricular mass and left ventricular mass indexed for body surface area (Table I).

Table 1: Left ventricular mass and blood pressure in children and adolescents.

Reference	BP	Age	BP/C	LVM	LVMI
Laird et al 1981	>95th	15	50/50	?	↑
Zahka et al 1981	>90th	8-19	61/49	↑	?
Hansen et al 1992 a	≧95th	9-11	64/66	↑	↑
Schieken et al 1981	>80th	9-18	111/153	↑	↑
Nishio et al 1986	>80th	9-12	31/32	↑	↑
Radice et al 1986	BH	14-19	25/55	↑	↑
Burke et al 1987	-	7-22	654	↑	NS

BP=blood pressure group; C=control group; BP/C=number; LVM=left ventricular mass; LVMI=LVM indexed for body surface area; ?=data not reported; ↑=increased; NS=not significant; BH=borderline hypertensives;

Familial relationships of high blood pressure levels have been documented in several pediatric population studies (Shear et al 1986). Although results from echocardiographic studies of left ventricular mass in offspring of hypertensives are controversial (Table II), the reported data suggest that cardiac involvement may precede clinically detectable hypertension, reflecting either a genetic predisposition to increased left ventricular mass or stimulation of left ventricular muscle growth by features not assessed by conventional blood pressure measurements. It has also been demonstrated that an increased left ventricular mass seems to be an important predictor of future blood pressure and subsequent hypertension (Mahoney et al 1988).

Physical fitness and blood pressure

An inverse correlation between blood pressure and physical fitness in adults is well-known (Blair et al 1984). In children, an inverse correlation between blood

Table 2: Left ventricular mass in offspring of hypertensives

Reference	Age	H/C	LVM	LVMI
Riopel et al 1980	10-17	68/52	↑	?
Radice et al 1986	14-19B	51/55	?	↑
de Leonardis et al 1988	14	14/15	?	NS
Graettinger et al 1988	12-15	21/26	NS	NS
Hansen et al 1992 b	9-11	43/64	NS	NS

H/C = number (offspring/control); LVM = left ventricular mass; LVMI = LVM indexed for body surface area; B = only males; ? = data not reported; ↑ = increased; NS = not significant.

pressure and physical fitness has also been demonstrated (Table III) (page 94), whether physical fitness was determined by submaximal (Fraser et al 1983, Hofman et al 1987, Panico et al 1987, Sallis et al 1988, Gutin et al 1990), or maximum (Wilson et al 1985, Hansen et al 1990) exercise approaches. However, an association between blood pressure and physical fitness, independent of differences in confounding variables including body size, has only been demonstrated for the submaximal approach. Other approaches for assessment of physical fitness, however, such as time required to complete a one mile run (Melby et al 1987) or performance time for a 20 m shuttle run test (Jenner et al 1992) did not correlate with blood pressure. Methodological problems inherent in assessment of physical fitness exist, and might explain some of the discrepant findings. Maximum oxygen uptake (in ml O_2 x min^{-1} x kg^{-1}) is probably the best approach to the assessment of physical fitness (Aastrand and Rodahl 1986).

Physical training and blood pressure

Physical training offers a potential non-pharmacological strategy for management of mild and borderline hypertension (World Hypertension League 1991). Most of the longitudinal training studies reviewed, however, must be interpreted with caution because of inadequate design, principally the absence of adequate and randomised control groups receiving the same care during the training period (Shephard 1992).

In children, attempts at educational intervention programmes that include recommendations on diet and physical activity alone (Puska et al 1982, Tell and Vellar 1987, Walter et al 1988) have not successfully controlled hypertension. A general approach combining low levels of drug treatment with an educational program directed towards hypertension and dietary and exercise modification (Berenson et al 1990) significantly reduced blood pressure in hypertensive children after 30 months of observation.

Table IV (page 95) shows the effect of physical training programmes on blood pressure and physical fitness in children. A controlled study of eight months of physical training with three extra lessons a week as part of an ordinary school physical education programme (Hansen et al 1991) significantly lowered blood pressure and improved physical fitness in both a normotensive training group and

Table 3: Blood pressure and physical fitness in children

Reference	Characteristics of study population			Major conclusions regarding blood pressure
	Age±SD	n	Source	
Fraser et al 1983	7-17	228	Selected sample of s.c., Southern California, USA	Univariate inverse correlation between PF and SBP/DBP
				Multivariate inverse correlation between PF and SBP (#DBP)
Wilson et al 1985	I:14±? C:14±?	102 90	Selected sample of s.c., Texas, USA	PF lower in girls (#boys) with BP ≥ 95th percentile
Hofman et al 1987	9±0.6	2061	Selected sample of s.c., New York, USA	Univariate and multivariate inverse correlation between PF and SBP/DBP
Panico et al 1987	7-14	1341	Sample of s.c., Naples, Italy	Univariate inverse correlation between PF and SBP (#DBP)
				Multivariate inverse correlation between PF and SBP in boys
Melby et al 1987	9-12	323	Sample of s.c., Indiana, USA	No correlation between PF and SBP/DBP
Sallis et al 1988	12	290	Selected sample of s.c., San Diego, USA	Univariate inverse correlation between PF and SBP/DBP
				Multivariate inverse correlation between PF and DBP in boys
Gutin et al 1990	5-6	216	Mainly ped. outpatients New York, USA	Univariate inverse correlation between PF and DBP (#SBP)
Hansen et al 1990	8-10	1284	Population of s.c., Odense, Denmark	Univariate inverse correlation between PF and SBP/DBP
				No multivariate correlation between PF and SBP/DBP
Jenner et al 1992	11-12	1092	Population of s.c., Perth, Australia	No correlation between PF and SBP/DBP
Dwyer et al 1994	9-15	2400	Selected sample of s.c., Australia	Univariate and multivariate inverse correlation between PF and SBP (#DBP)

SD=standard deviation; n=number; s.c.=schoolchildren; I=index group; C=control group; BP=blood pressure; SBP=systolic BP; DBP=diastolic BP; PF=physical fitness; ?=data not reported; #=but not

a hypertensive training group, compared with changes in the controls. Three months of training did not significantly change either blood pressure or physical fitness. Four months of physical training in 11-13 year old boys did not change blood pressure (Eriksson and Koch 1973), and although physical fitness increased significantly after eight weeks (Linder et al 1983) and fourteen weeks (Dwyer et al 1983) of physical training, no changes could be demonstrated in blood pressure. A significant decrease in both systolic and diastolic blood pressure and a simultaneous increase in physical fitness have been observed after six months of training (Hagberg et al 1983). A 20-week weight loss program combining exercise and caloric restriction in obese children significantly reduced blood pressure, but no changes could be demonstrated in physical fitness (Rocchini et al 1988).

Table 4: Effects of dynamic training on blood pressure and physical fitness in children

Reference	Characteristics of study population			Training program				Blood pressure (mm Hg)				Change in PF
	Age		n	Methods	Frequency (per week)	Time (min)	Duration	Systolic BP Pre	Post	Diastolic BP Pre	Post	(%)
Eriksson and Koch 1973	11-13B	T	9	Bicycle	3	60	4 mo	?	$NS	?	$NS	+19#
Dwyer et al 1983	10.2±?	T	172	HR(I) every s.day	75		14 we	102.0	100.8	63.4	59.6	+23#
		S	185	HR(0) every s.day	75		14 we	102.6	101.4	63.1	58.4	+16
		C	162	-	-	-	14 we	103.0	101.9	62.3	60.8	+11
Hagberg et al 1983	14-18	T	25	Jogging	5	30-40	6 mo	137	129#	80	75#	+10#
		D		-	-	-	9 mo	139		78		0
Linder et al 1983	11-17B	T	29	Jogging	3	30	8 we	103.6	102.3	62.4	64.9	+15*#
		C	21	-	-	-		99.0	100.8	62.1	62.7	-1
Rocchini et al 1988	10-17	T+D	25	Aerobic/diet	3	60	20 we	129	113*	79	66*	+2
		+D	26	Diet	1	60	20 we	127	117*	80	68*	-8
		C	22	-	-	-	-	126	130	78	77	0
Hansen et al 1991	9-11	T	67	Sch.phys.	3	45	8 mo	108	104*	71	71*	+5*
		C	65	-	-	-	8 mo	111	111	73	76	-1
Vandongen et al 1995	10-12	T	81	Sch.phys. ev.s.day		15	9 mo	103.6	100.5	60.9	56.0	+12*#
		C	67	-	-	-	9 mo	105.9	103.1	61.1	57.9	-3

PF=physical fitness; n=number; BP=blood pressure; B=only boys; T=training group; C=control group; D=detraining group; +D=diet and behavior change; HR(I)=activities which intended to rise heart rate: HR(0)=skilled activities which did not intend to rise; heart rate; s.=school; Sch.phys.=school physical education program; we=week; mo=month; ?=data not reported; *P<0.05 or less (T vs C); #P<0.05 or less (pre vs post); NS=not significant; $=change during activity period

The mechanisms responsible for the blood pressure lowering effect of physical training are unknown. The time course dependency implies that the adaptive responses to physical training occurs rather slowly over a prolonged period of time. Irrespective of which mechanism might be involved, it includes, possibly, multiple adaptive reactions occurring primarily in the skeletal muscle fibres, in the nervous system, and in the circulatory system (Clausen 1977).

The long-term course of blood pressure in children after a physical training program is unknown. An inverse relationship between 1-year and 5-year changes in children's physical fitness and changes in blood pressure has been reported (Hofman and Walter 1989). A very substantial cardiovascular benefit might result from a 3 mm Hg (Rose 1981) or a 5 mm Hg (Wilkins and Calabrese 1985) reduction in the blood pressure of the entire population, and physical training is a strategy by which this kind of population-wide blood pressure reduction could be achieved.

Physical training, therefore, might prove effective as an important non-pharmacological approach to primary prevention of essential hypertension. Therefore, the encouragement of children to participate in physical training programmes scheduled with at least three sessions per week for at least 30 minutes per session at 60-70 % of individual maximal oxygen uptake is strongly recommended.

References

Barker DJP, Gluckman PD, Godfrey KM, Harding JE, Owens JA, Robinson JS. Fetal nutrition and cardiovascular disease in adult life. Lancet 1993;341:938-41.

Berenson GS, Shear CL, Chiang YK, Webber LS, Voors AW. Combined low-dose medication and primary intervention over a 30-month period for sustained high blood pressure in childhood. Am J Med Sci 1990;299:79-86.

Berenson GS, Wattiigney WA, Bao W, Nicklas TA, Jiang X, Rush JA. Epidemiology of early primary hypertension and implications for prevention: The Bogalusa Heart Study. J Hum Hypertens 1994;8:303-11.

Blair SN, Goodyear NN, Gibbons LW, Cooper KH. Physical fitness and incidence of hypertension in healthy normotensive men and women. JAMA 1984;252:487-90.

Burke GL, Arcilla RA, Culpepper WS, Webber LS, Chiang YK, Berenson GS. Blood pressure and echocardiographic measures in children: the Bogalusa Heart Study. Circulation 1987;1:106-14.

Clausen JP. Effect of physical training on cardiovascular adjustments to exercise in man. Physiol Rev 1977;57:779-815.

de Man SA, André JL, Bachmann H, Grobbee DE, Ibsen KK, Laaser U, Lippert P, Hofman A. Blood pressure in childhood: Pooled findings of six European studies. J Hypertens 1991;9:109-14.

De Leonardis V, De Scalzi M, Falchette A, Cinelli P, Croppi E, Livi R, Scarpelli L, Scarpelli PT. Echocardiographic evaluation of children with and without family history of essential hypertension. Am J Hypertens 1988;1:305-8.

Devereux RB. Importance of left ventricular mass as a predictor of cardiovascular morbidity in hypertension. Am J Hypertens 1989;2:650-4.

Dwyer T, Coonan WE, Leitch DR, Hetzel BS, Baghurst RA. An investigation of the effects of daily physical activity on the health of primary school students in South Australia. Int J Epidemiol 1983;12:308-13.

Eriksson BO, Koch G. Effect of physical training on hemodynamic response during submaximal and maximal exercise in 11-13-year old boys. Acta Physiol Scand 1973;87:27-39.

Fraser GE, Phillips RL, Harris R. Physical fitness and blood pressure in school children. Circulation 1983;67:405-12.

Graettinger WF, Cheung DE, Lipson JL, Hoffman CA, Weber MA. Correlates of cardiac structure and function in normotensive adolescents. Am J Hypertens 1988;1:184-6.

Gutin B, Basch C, Shea S, Contento I, DeLozier M, Rips J, Irigoyen M, Zybert P. Blood pressure, fitness, and fatness in 5- and 6-year-old children. JAMA 1990;264:1123-7.

Hagberg JM, Goldring D, Ehsani AA, Heath GW, Hernandez A, Schechtman K, Holloszy JO. Effect of exercise training on the blood pressure and hemodynamic features of hypertensive adolescents. Am J Cardiol 1983;52:763-8.

Hansen HS, Froberg K, Hyldebrandt N, Nielsen JR. A controlled study of eight months of physical training and reduction of blood pressure in children: The Odense Schoolchild Study. Br Med J 1991;303:682-5.

Hansen HS, Hyldebrandt N, Froberg K, Nielsen JR. Blood pressure and physical fitness in a population of children - the Odense Schoolchild Study. J Hum Hypertens 1990;4:615-20.

Hansen HS, Nielsen JR, Froberg K, Hyldebrandt N. Left ventricular hypertrophy in children from the upper five percent of the blood pressure distribution – The Odense Schoolchild Study. J Hum Hypertens 1992 a;6:41-5.

Hansen HS, Nielsen JR, Hyldebrandt N, Froberg K. Blood pressure and cardiac structure in children with a parental history of hypertension: The Odense Schoolchild Study. J Hypertens 1992 b;10:677-82.

Hofman A, Walter HJ, Connelly PA, Vaughan RD. Blood pressure and physical fitness in children. Hypertension 1987;9:188-91.

Hofman A, Walter HJ. The association between physical fitness and cardiovascular disease risk factors in children in a five-year follow-up study. Int J Epidemiol 1989;18:830-5.

Jenner DA, Vandongen R, Beilin L. Relationships between blood pressure and measures of dietary energy intake, physical fitness, and physical activity in Australian children aged 11-12 years. J Epidemiol Community Health 1992;46:108-13.

Koren MJ, Devereux RB, Casale PN, Savage DD, Laragh JH. Relation of left ventricular mass and geometry to morbidity and mortality in uncomplicated essential hypertension. Ann Intern Med 1991;114:345-52.

Laird WP, Fixler DE. Left ventricular hypertrophy in adolescents with elevated blood pressure: assessment by chest roentgenography, electrocardiography, and echocardiography. Pediatrics 1981;67:255-9.

Lever AF, Harrap SB. Essential hypertension: A disorder of growth with origins in childhood? J Hypertens 1992;10:101-20.

Linder CW, DuRant RH, Mahoney OM. The effect of physical conditioning on serum lipids and lipoproteins in white male adolescents. Med Sci Sports Exerc 1983;15:232-6.

Mahoney LT, Schieken RM, Clarke WR, Lauer RM. Left ventricular mass and exercise responses predict future blood pressure. The Muscatine Study. Hypertension 1988;12:206-13.

Melby CL, Dunn PJ, Hyner GC, Sedlock D, Corrigan DL. Correlates of blood pressure in elementary schoolchildren. J Sch Health 1987;57:375-8.

Nishio T, Mori C, Saito M, Haneda N, Kajino Y, Watanabe K, Suzuki K. Tracking of blood pressure, height, weight and left ventricular muscle volume in children-the Shimane Heart Study. Jpn Circ J 1986;50:1321-4.

Panico S, Celentano E, Krogh V, Jossa F, Farinaro E, Trevisan M, Mancini M. Physical activity and its relationship to blood pressure in school children. J Chronic Dis 1987; 40:925-30.

Puska P, Vartiainen E, Pallonen U, Salonen JT, Pöyhiä P, Koskela K, McAlister A. The North Karelia Youth Project: Evaluation of two years of intervention on health behavior and CVD risk factors among 13- to 15-year-old children. Prev Med 1982;11:550-70.

Radice M, Alli C, Avanzini F, Di Tullio M, Mariotti G, Taioli E, Zussino A, Folli G. Left ventricular structure and function in normotensive adolescents with a genetic predisposition to hypertension. Am Heart J 1986;111:115-20.

Report of the Second Task Force on Blood Pressure Control in Children-1987. Pediatrics 1987;79:1-25.

Riopel DA, Hohn AR, Taylor AB, Loadholt BC. Echocardiographic variables in progeny of hypertensive and normotensive parents. Circulation 1980;62(suppl III):270.

Rocchini AP, Katch V, Anderson J, Hinderliter J, Becque D, Martin M, Marks C. Blood pressure in obese adolescents: effect of weight loss. Pediatrics 1988;82:16-23.

Rose G. Strategy of prevention: Lessons from cardiovascular disease. Br Med J 1981; 282:1847-51.

Sallis JF, Patterson TL, Buono MJ, Nader PR. Relation of cardiovascular fitness and physical activity to cardiovascular disease risk factors in children and adults. Am J Epidemiol 1988;127:933-41.

Schieken RM, Clarke WR, Lauer RM. Left ventricular hypertrophy in children with blood pressures in the upper quintile of the distribution: The Muscatine Study. Hypertension 1981;3:669-75.

Shear CL, Burke GL, Freedman DS, Berenson GS. Value of childhood blood pressure measurements and family history in predicting future blood pressure status: results from 8 years of follow-up in the Bogalusa Heart Study. Pediatrics 1986;77:862-9.

Shephard RJ. Effectiveness of training programmes for prepubescent children. Sports Med 1992;13:194-213.

Tell GS, Vellar OD. Noncommunicable disease risk factor intervention in Norwegian adolescents: the Oslo youth study. In: Hetzel BS, Berenson GS, eds. Cardiovascular risk factors in childhood: epidemiology and prevention. Amsterdam: Elsevier, 1987:203-17.

Vandongen R, Jenner DA, Thompson C, Taggart AC, Spickett EE, Burke V, Beilin LJ, Milligan RA, Dunbar DL. A controlled evaluation of a fitness and nutrition intervention program on cardiovascular health in 10- to 12-year-old children. Prev Med 1995;24:9-22.

Walter HJ, Hofman A, Vaughan AD, Wynder EL. Modification of risk factors for coronary heart disease. N Engl J Med 1988;318:1093-1100.

Wilkins III JR, Calabrese EJ. Health implications of a 5 mm Hg increase in blood pressure. Toxicol Ind Health 1985;1:13-28.

Wilson SL, Gaffney FA, Laird WP, Fixler DE. Body size, composition, and fitness in adolescents with elevated blood pressures. Hypertension 1985;7:417-22.

World Hypertension League. Physical exercise in the management of hypertension: A consensus statement by the World Hypertension League. J Hypertens 1991;9:283-7.

Zahka KG, Neill CA, Kidd L, Cutilletta MA, Cutilletta AF. Cardiac involvement in adolescent hypertension: Echocardiographic determination of myocardial hypertrophy. Hypertension 1981;3:664-8.

Aastrand PO, Rodahl K, editors. Textbook of work physiology. 3rd ed., New York: McGraw-Hill Book Company, 1986:354-90.

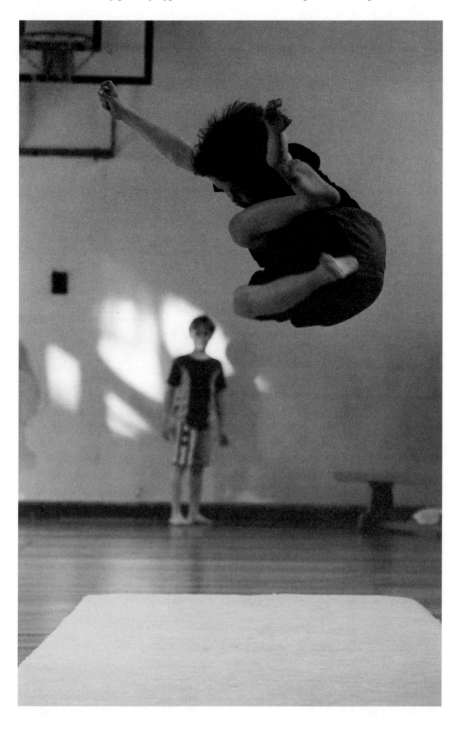

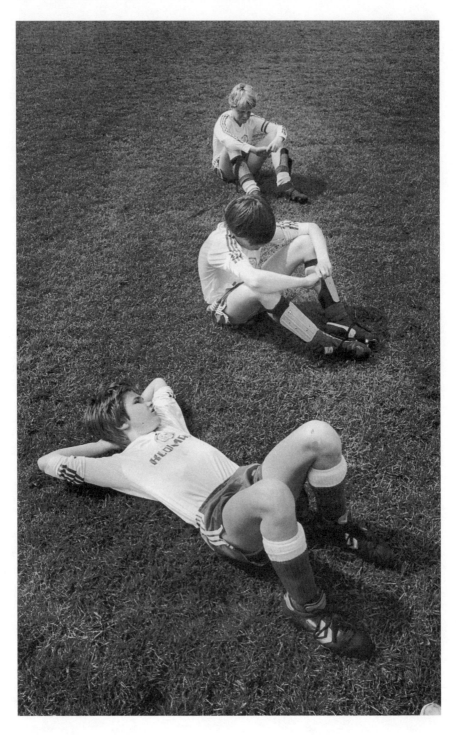

Chapter 8

Unexpected Sudden Death From Heart Disease in the Young

Frank M. Galioto

The unexpected death of a child, adolescent or young adult is a tragedy without parallel in man's experience. These unexpected deaths are felt by family, friends, and, indeed, by society itself and raise significant questions as to the general well-being and health of all young individuals. Many of these deaths are avoidable as they occur in patients with known congenital heart disease who are engaged in inappropriate activities. But others should be considered inevitable, even if the diagnosis has been made, given the nature of the diseases involved and the ultimate poor prognosis associated with those diseases.

In this paper, I will discuss the main cardiovascular causes of sudden death in the young and also discuss possible modes of prevention. The incidence of unexpected cardiac death in children is low. In the large Mayo Clinic series, the rate was 1.3 cases per 100,000 patient years.[1] A study by McCafree[2] revealed that five of 100,000 young athletes may have a condition which places them at risk for sudden death but only 1 in 200,000 actually die. It is obvious from these numbers that large population studies, which are very difficult to conduct because of problems in obtaining complete reporting of patients with sudden death and the lack of complete and accurate autopsy findings, are at best estimates, but it is clear that the incidence is low.[3]

A study done on young recruits in the Israeli Army reported ten sudden deaths related to exercise in 12 years.[4] Fifty percent of these were thought to be due to heart disease and 16.7 percent were without an identified cause based on the autopsy. These additional 16.7 percent of patients may well have died of arrhythmia as those patients often have a structurally normal heart. Looking at the 20 sudden deaths, it was important to recognize that 40% had prior syncope and 30% had prior chest pain.

For this presentation, the etiologies of sudden cardiac death in the young will be divided into seven categories: Hypertrophic cardiomyopathy, coronary artery abnormalities, structural defects of the heart, arrhythmias, inflammatory disease, atherosclerotic coronary artery disease and connective tissue diseases. Each of these will be addressed in turn with emphasis on diagnosis and possible mechanism of death.

Hypertrophic cardiomyopathy

Hypertrophic cardiomyopathy is the leading cause of sudden and unexpected death in young athletes .[5] It often occurs without preceding symptoms and unfortunately, its prevalence is relatively high at one per 1,000 general population. The disease is often silent on physical examination but can easily be diagnosed by echocardiography. Hypertrophic cardiomyopathy has an autosomal dominant inheritance pattern with variable penetrance in half of the cases.[6] In the other half, it is considered to be sporadic mutation. Currently, at least seven gene loci have been identified as causes of hypertrophic cardiomyopathy. The annual mortality for patients with the disease is considered to be 1%, but in selected families, it is 2.4% and, unfortunately, in younger patients, is as high as 6%. It is felt that the younger patients may be at higher risk because they are engaged in more stressful activities which makes them more prone to develop the mechanisms which lead to sudden death.

Hypertrophic cardiomyopathy is characterized by a massive thickening of the myocardium of the left ventricle, often in an asymmetric pattern with thickening of the interventricular septum predominating. The right ventricle is often slightly thickened but it is the abnormalities of the septal and left ventricular free walls that characterizes the disease. On echocardiography, this is easily recognized as is a characteristic systolic anterior movement of the mitral valve. Left ventricular outflow is obstructed because of the septal hypertrophy and the motion of the mitral valve so that in midsystole, instead of having a normal rise in the ventricular pressure, there is a steeper rise with a fall in aortic flow with the increasing obstruction. This obstruction in midsystole results in a bisferiens pulse with a double hump felt in the peripheral pulse.

The mechanisms of sudden death in hypertrophic cardiomyopathy are thought to be ventricular dysrhythmia, atrial dysrhythmia and myocardial ischemia.[7] Ventricular arrhythmia is thought to arise because the patients have an increased mass of the myocardium without concomitant increase in myocardial perfusion. This mismatch is aggravated by the obstruction of outflow into the aortic root, therefore decreasing coronary perfusion to significant areas of afterloaded ventricular myocardium. In periods of increased cardiac output such as sports, this mismatch can become critical with very inadequate blood flow to the myocardium. A second mode of death is thought to be due to atrial fibrillation with rapid ventricular response. This has been recognized as a cause for some years but it is much less common than the ventricular dysrhythmia mode. Some patients are thought to have myocardiac ischemia without ventricular dysrhythmia because of the increased mass of the myocardium and the lack of adequate blood supply. This is aggravated during exercise with resultant ischemia which may, in turn, predispose to ventricular dysrhythmias. Ventricular tachycardia can develop which then rapidly degenerates into ventricular fibrillation and death. All of these mechanisms are interrelated and all are worsened by increased activity.

Clinical predictors of sudden death in hypertrophic cardiomyopathy include left ventricular hypertrophy on the electrocardiogram, a family history of sudden death, age of the patient with the younger patients at higher risk, the degree of left ventricular outflow tract obstruction, myocardial ischemia on resting or exercise electro-cardiograms, prior history of cardiac arrest and known ventricular tachycardia.[6] Un-fortunately, the majority of patients have no clinical symptoms prior to a sudden death episode. In younger patients, syncope related to exercise may be a warning sign. Holter monitoring is not as useful in young patients as it is in older individuals as arrhythmia at rest is not as common a feature in the younger patients.

Sudden death may be delayed but not necessarily prevented in these patients. Exercise modification is useful but often the activities of daily living call for sud-den stressful activity which may predispose to ventricular dysrhythmias. A number of pharmacological agents have been tried and while they do not prevent sudden death, they may alleviate symptoms. These include beta-blockers and calcium channel blockers. These drugs have been used extensively in children and while they may increase the longevity of the patient, they are not felt to necessarily pre-vent sudden death. Surgical myotomy and myectomy of the septum and left ven-tricular outflow tract again may relieve symptoms but these operations have been shown not to prevent death in these patients. Implantable defibrillators and dual chamber pacemakers are current therapies under evaluation. They have again been useful in improving the day-to-day status of the patient but have not been shown to prevent sudden death. Many believe that gene therapy in the future is a potential mode of therapy but unfortunately this is still theoretical.

Coronary artery anomalies

Coronary artery anomalies represent another major cause of sudden death. The study by Virmani et al. included an autopsy study of 242 patients.[9] Anomalous ori-gin of the left coronary artery from the right sinus of valsalva and origin of the right coronary artery from the left sinus were most commonly related to sudden death. Younger patients were much more likely to die suddenly and during activity. In these coronary artery abnormalities, a coronary artery arises abnormally from the aortic root and passes between the aorta and the pulmonary artery. For ex-ample, if the right and left coronary arteries both arise from the right sinus of val-salva, the course of the left coronary artery may go anteriorly between the aorta which is posterior and to the right and the pulmonary artery which is anterior and to the left. At rest, when the pulmonary artery pressure is low and there is no in-creased myocardial oxygen demand, coronary flow is adequate. With activity which will increase both pulmonary artery pressure and pulmonary artery size as well as the myocardial oxygen demands, the left coronary artery is compressed between the aorta and the pulmonary artery therefore reducing coronary blood flow at that time of peak demands. This compression results in myocardial ische-mia which predisposes to arhythmia and sudden death. Patients with this anomaly often have angina-like pain during exercise.

The diagnosis of a coronary artery origin abnormality can often be made by echocardiography where the origins of the coronary arteries are identified in the short axis view and then confirmed by angiography. Coronary bypass or relocation of the origin of the anomalous coronary artery to another sinus is curative in these patients.

Structural heart disease

A third group at risk for sudden death are patients with structural heart disease. The most common lesion associated with sudden death is aortic stenosis of all types including subvalve, valvar and supravalvar obstructions. Eisenmenger's complex with pulmonary vascular obstructive disease comprised the next most common in the Lambert study[10] but the sum of these two lesions did not constitute the majority of cases with a variety of other lesions implicated. By analyzing the patients' activities at the time of their death, many were clearly engaged in inappropriate activity. These unfortunate children had either disregarded the advice of their cardiologist as to what activity was prohibited, or had not had adequate direction from their cardiologist.

Another important structural defect of the heart not included in the original Lambert Study which is silent on physical exam but a significant cause of sudden death, is arrhythogenic right ventricular dysplasia.[11] This is an autosomal dominant syndrome with variable penetrance. In these patients, the myocardium of the ventricle is thinned and dysplastic and prone to the development of significant dysrhythmias including ventricular tachycardia which may degenerate into ventricular fibrillation. Treatment with beta-blockers has proven to be helpful in some cases but it remains to be proven if that mode of therapy will prevent sudden death in the long-term.

Arrhythmia

Another significant causative group is sudden death from arrhythmia. Within this group, I will discuss five major types of dysrhythmia: Prolonged QT syndrome, postoperative arrhythmias, Wolff-Parkinson-White syndrome, congenital heart block and ventricular tachyarrhythmias with a structurally normal heart.

The prolonged QT syndrome has been recognized for many years as being associated with sudden and unexpected death.[12] The patients have a structurally normal heart, therefore having no findings on a resting physical examination. An international study of 287 patients revealed the hallmark of the lesion to be a corrected QT interval on the electrocardiogram of greater than 0.44 seconds. In this disorder, the prolonged repolarization leads to torsades de pointes, a form of ventricular tachycardia. Most patients had a history of unexplained syncope, seizures or cardiac arrest. Often, there is a family history of prolonged QT syndrome and the mean age of presentation for this large group was 6.8 years. The Villain study from France[13] examined 15 neonates with the long QT syndrome who had developed symptoms. Eight had QT intervals greater than 0.60 seconds and all of these patients developed severe ventricular dysrhythmias. Twelve of the 15 patients were treated with betablockers but four died despite therapy and pacing. Of the 15 patients, five had normalization of their QT interval after one year of age.

In our group's experience with prolonged QT syndrome, 67% of the patients developed symptoms from arrhythmia related to exercise. Thirty-nine percent of our patients had a family history positive for a prolonged QT and a family history positive for sudden death in 31%. Only 4.5% of patients had congenital deafness. The

Pediatric Electrophysiology Society study of 287 patients[14] revealed that patients with atrial ventricular block, multiform premature ventricular beats, QT intervals greater than 0.60 seconds and torsade were at highest risk. Patients who had a prolonged QT but were asymptomatic should always be treated initially with beta-blockers. If this mode of therapy does not correct their QT interval, patients must go on to a left stellate ganglion resection or implantable defibrillators.

A subgroup of this group of patients are those with iatrogenic prolonged QT interval caused by increasing use of medications which alter cardiac repolarization. The most common class of drugs that produce this prolongation are the tricyclic medications which are used for behavior. Ventricular fibrillation can be produced in these patients by altering repolarization. Therefore, a screening electrocardiogram is needed for all patients on the tricyclic class of medications.

Postoperative congenital heart disease patients are known to have significant dysrhythmias, especially patients after repair of tetralogy of Fallot,[15] transposition after atrial switch procedures,[16] and Fontan patients.[17] In these patients, the surgical repair has either caused isolated ventricular myocardial damage or has altered the normal pathways which conduct the impulses through the heart. Sudden death following repair of tetralogy of Fallot has been greatly reduced by careful monitoring of patients for signs of ventricular dysrhythmias and assuring that the hemodynamic repair is adequate. Patients with Mustard's and Senning's repair in our practice have a 10% incidence of sick sinus syndrome per year after this type of repair and many go on to require pacemakers. If these children develop sinus node or AV node block during exercise, they could have sudden induction of low heart rates during peak exercise and may be prone to development of other dysrhythmias or sudden death. Finally, the patients who have had Fontan's operation with connections of the systemic venous return directly to the lungs and bypassing an obstructed right heart commonly develop atrial flutter because of extensive surgery done in the right atrium. These patients may develop atrial flutter and an altered conduction system may make their single ventricular chamber more susceptible to the development of ventricular tachycardia and fibrillation.

Patients with Wolff-Parkinson-White syndrome or ventricular preexcitation are also at risk for sudden death.[18] This risk is especially true in patients with either short antegrade refractory periods of their accessory connection or patients who are on digoxin which may block their normal conduction pathways. Any patient with a short antegrade refractory period who develops an atrial tachyarrhythmia will have a very high ventricular rate in response which will predispose to ventricular tachycardia and ventricular fibrillation. Currently, therapy for these patients with catheter ablation may be life saving.

Patients with complete congenital heart block are known to develop ventricular ectopy, syncope and congestive heart failure.[19] All of these, plus exercise intolerance, are indications for pacemaker implantation. Most cardiologists who care for patients with congenital complete heart block believe that pacemaker implantation may be lifesaving if any ventricular ectopy or symptoms develop.

Finally, patients may develop sudden death from arrythmia without having structural heart disease or other anatomic substrates. Benson, in a study of 11 patients, aged 15 months to 29 years, who had survived sudden death episodes by prompt resuscitation found at electrophysiologic study that eight of these patients had inducible sustained tachycardia. Six of the eight had ventricular tachycardia; one had supraventricular tachycardia and one had atrial flutter with concealed pre-excitation of the WPW variety. Despite a series of therapeutic interventions, three patients with ventricular tachycardia went on to die despite all efforts. Further studies of patients with ventricular arrhythmias have identified the subset of patients with a dilated left ventricle and cardiomyopathy to be at more significant risk for arrhythmia and sudden death. If the primary problem is a dilated cardiomyopathy, treatment of the dysrhythmia with pharmacologic agents and implantable defibrillators may be of assistance in preventing sudden death as would a modification of activity. It is not proven, however, that these patients will have long-term survivability because of the progressive nature of their cardiac dilatation and cardiomyopathy. Finally, in an interesting study by Furanello[21], 766 patients with exercises symptoms were studied and 31 were found to have ventricular dysrhythmias. Athletic activity was found to be a trigger of electrical destabilization in these patients. The role of electrophysiologic studies for these patients was unclear, however, as in many, the ventricular dysrhythmia could not be induced during electrophysiologic study but only during athletic induction.

Inflammatory diseases

Inflammatory diseases are considered rarer but recognizable causes of sudden death in young athletes. An overwhelming myocarditis is considered to be an uncommon but recognizable cause of sudden death. The etiology of the myocarditis is usually viral and therapy is still controversial. Recent studies have shown no statistical benefit from steroid or anti-inflammatory agents during the period of the acute inflammation.[22] General support and treatment of any symptoms of congestive heart failure are obviously recommended. In very small children, bacterial sepsis should always be considered as a cause of a myocarditis. Myocarditis is often difficult to separate from a dilated cardiomyopathy and endomyocardial biopsy is recommended. The prognosis for myocarditis is felt to be better than that of a dilated cardiomyopathy with myocarditis having a shorter course and more amenable to anticongestive heart failure therapies.

Another important inflammatory process which can cause sudden death in a very young patient is Kawasaki's disease.[23] Early recognition of this disorder which has no known etiology, as well as prompt treatment with immunoglobulins reduces the incidence of complicating features and of death. Eighteen percent of patients in our practice with Kawasaki's disease developed coronary artery aneurysms before the institution of immunoglobulin therapy. The death rate was between 1% and 3%. With immunoglobulin therapy in the first 10 days of the disease, the incidence of aneurysms is slightly less than 10% and the risk of sudden death is less than 1%. Recent work has shown that many years after the acute phase of the Kawasaki's disease, there may be late ischemia of the myocardium by radionuclide assessment on stress testing. It may well be that the coronary artery inflammation found in these patients may produce early coronary stenosis which can predispose to premature atherosclerotic disease in early adulthood.[24]

Atherosclerotic coronary disease

Sudden death from premature atherosclerotic coronary artery disease in itself is very rare in patients less than 21 years of age in all studies including patients with abnormal lipid profiles.[25] However, it is believed that treatment of abnormal lipid metabolism during childhood and adolescence may lessen the incidence of premature coronary artery disease in young adults. The nature of the treatment of these lipid disorders is controversial but often a simple diet and increased exercise is most useful in reducing total cholesterol and increasing HDL cholesterol.

Connective tissue diseases

Connective tissue diseases are important but uncommon causes of sudden death in young individuals. Marfan's disease is the most common category in this group. This is an autosomal dominant disease with variable penetrance. The cardiovascular manifestations of Marfan's disease include aortic root dilatation with possible rupture of the aorta during exercise due to increased aortic wall tension. Mitral valve prolapse is always present, usually with mitral regurgitation. It has been shown by several investigators that treatment with beta-blockers is effective in slowing the progression of the disease. Only appropriate activities must be permitted for patients with Marfan's syndrome with avoidance of isometrics which would increase blood pressure and lateral wall tension on the abnormal vessels.

The issue of isolated mitral valve prolapse, a common disorder, is quite controversial. Most investigators feel that mitral valve prolapse is not associated with sudden death in young individuals. However, Dollar and Roberts[27] found mitral prolapse as the only pathologic finding at autopsy in 15 patients who had an average age of 39 years. That study could not exclude arrhythmia as an independent risk factor. Further studies are clearly required to identify the association of sudden death and mitral prolapse. Currently, patients with mitral valve prolapse, without regurgitation and those with only mild regurgitation are permitted full activities in our practice.

Prevention

The prevention of sudden cardiac death should always be part of the evaluation of any athlete. Athletes who present with exercise-related syncope and chest pain deserve further evaluation as do patients with a family history of unexplained sudden death, Marfan's disease, hypertrophic cardiomyopathy and prolonged QT syndrome. Similarly, all patients with congenital heart disease need to be carefully evaluated before they are allowed to participate in athletics so that events that are safe for them are permitted and those that are not safe are not permitted.

Studies that may be used in a prevention program for diagnosis include a careful history and physical examination, resting electrocardiogram, echocardiogram, stress testing and, in some cases, a genetic assessment. The question of who should receive this extensive and rather expensive evaluation is a societal question rather than one for the cardiologist. If all children receive electrocardiograms, echocardiograms and stress testing, we can certainly reduce the incidence of sudden death during sports from previously undiagnosed disorders. A human genome analysis for all patients may lead to certain other patients who are at risk. Certainly, modification of diet and better physical activities for all patients is always recommended.

The selection of the correct activity for the patient with known heart disease is always the responsibility of the treating cardiologist. If a child dies during sports that were approved by the cardiologist, there has been an error in management. If the child disregards the advice of the cardiologist and is permitted by his family to engage in inappropriate activities, the cardiologist is not directly at fault but one should always strive for better educational efforts for the patient and family so that they are less likely to engage in inappropriate activities.

References

1. Driscoll. D.J. and Edwards. W.D.: Sudden Unexpected Death in Children and Adolescents. J. Am Coll Cardiol 5:118B. 1985.
2. McCaffrey. F.M.. Braden, D.S. and Strong. W.B.: Sudden Cardiac Death in Young Athletes. AJDC 145:177. 1991.
3. Waller. B.F., Hawley, D.A., Clark. M.A. and Pless. J.E.: Incidence of Sudden Athletic Deaths Between 1985 and 1990 In Marion County. Indiana. Clin Cardiol 15:851. 1992.
4. Kramer. M. R., Drori, Y. and Lev, B.: Sudden Death in Young Soldiers. Chest 93:345, 1988.
5. Maron. B.J., Spirito. P., Wesley, Y. and Arce, J.: Development and Progression of Left Ventricular Hypertrophy in Children with Hypertrophic Cardiomyopathy. N Engl J Med 315:610, 1986.
6. Marian. A.J.: Sudden Cardiac Death in Patients with Hypertrophic Cardiomyopathy: From Bench to Bedside with an Emphasis on Genetic Markers. Clin Cardiol 18:189, 1995.
7. McKenna. W.J., Camm, A.J.: Sudden Death in Hypertrophic Cardiomyopathy; Assessment of Patients at High Risk. Circ 80:1489, 1989.
8. Spirito. P., Chiarella, F., Carritino. L., Berisso, M.Z., Bellotti, P., and Vecchio, C.: Clinical Course and Prognosis of Hypertrophic Cardiomyopathy in an Outpatient Population. N Engl J Med 320:749, 1989.
9. Virmani, R., Rogan. K.. Cheitlin. M.D.: Congenital Coronary Artery Anomalies: Pathologic Aspects. In: Virmani, R., Forman, M.B. eds. Nonatherosclerotic Ischemic Heart Disease, New York: Raven Press, 1989 : 153 .
10. Lambert. E.C., Vijayan, A.M., Wagner, H.R., and Vlad, P.: Sudden Unexpected Death from Cardiovascular Disease in Children, A Cooperative International Study. Am J Cardiol 34:89, 1974.
11. Virmani. R., Robinowitz, M., Clark, M.A. and McAllister, H.A.: Sudden Death and Congenital Partial Absence of the Right Ventricular Myocardium: Arch Pathol Lab Med 106:163. 1982.
12. Moss, A.J., Schwartz, P.J., Crampton. R.S., Locati, E., and Carleen, E.: The Long QT Syndrome: A Prospective International Study. Circ 71:17. 1985.
13. Villain E., Levy. M., Kachaner, J., and Garson. A.: Prolonged QT Interval In Neonates: Benign, Transient, or Prolonged Risk of Sudden Death. Am Heart J 124:194, 1992.
14. Garson. A., Dick. M., Fournier, A: The Long QT Syndrome in Children: An International Study of 287 Patients. Circ 87:1866. 1993.
15. Gatzoulis. M.A., Till, J.A., Somerville, J., and Redington, A.N.: Mechanoelectric Interaction in Tetralogy of Fallot. Circ 92:231, 1995.

16. Graham. T.P.: Hemodynamic Residua and Sequelae Following Intra-Atrial Repair of Transposition of the Great Arteries: A Review. Pediatr Cardiol 2:203, 1982.
17. Driscoll. D.J.: Exercise Responses in Functional Single Ventricle Before and After Fontan Operation. Prog Pediatr Cardiol 2:44, 1993.
18. Munger. T.M., Packer, D.L., and Hammill, S.C.: A Population Study of the Natural History of Wolff-Parkinson-White Syndrome in Olmsted County, Minnesota 1953-1989. Circ 87:866, 1993.
19. Karpawich. P.P., Gillette, P.C., Garson, A., Hesslein, P.S., Porter, C B, and McNamara, D.G.: Congenital Complete Atrioventricular Block: Clinical and Electrophysiologic Predictors of Need for Pacemaker Insertion. Am J Cardiol 48:1098, 1981.
20. Benson, D.W., Benditt, D.G., Anderson, R.W., Dunnigan, A., Pritsker, M.R., Kulik, T.J., and Zavoral, J.H.: Cardiac Arrestin Young, Ostensibly Healthy Patients: Clinical, Hemodynamic, and Electrophysiologic Findings. Am J Cardiol 52:65, 1983.
21. Furlanello. F., Bertoldi, A., Bettini, R., Dallago, M., And Vergara, G.: Life-Threatening Tachyarrhythmias in Athletes. PACE 15:1403, 1992 .
22. Mason, J.W., O'Connell, J.B., Herskowitz, A., Rose, N.R., McManus, B.M., Billingham, M.E., and Moon, T.E.: A Clinical Trial of Immunosuppressive Therapy for Myocarditis. N Engl J Med 333:269,
23. Takahashi. M.: Inflammatory Disease of the Coronary Arteryin Children. Cor Art Dis 4:133. 1993.
24. Paridon. S.M., Galioto. F.M., Vincent, J.A., Tamassoni. T.L., Sullivan, N.M. and Bricher. J.T.: Exercise Capacity and Incidence of Myocardial Perfusion Defects After Kawasaki Disease in Children and Adolescents. J Am Coll Cardiol 25:1420. 1995.
25. Johnson, W.D., Strong. J.P., Oalmann. M., Newman, W.P., Tracy, R.E., and Rock, W.A.: Sudden Death From Coronary Heart Disease in Young Men. Arch Pathol Lab Med 105:227, 1981.
26. Maron. B.J., Roberts, W.C., McAllister, H.A., Rosing, D.R., and Epstein, S.E. Sudden Death in Young Athletes. Circ 62:218, 1980. 27.
    Dollar, A.L. and Roberts, W.C.: Morphologic Comparison of Patient with Mitral Valve Prolapse Who Died Suddenly with Patients Who Died From Severe Valvular Dysfunction or Other Conditions. J Am Coll Cardiol 17:921, 1991.

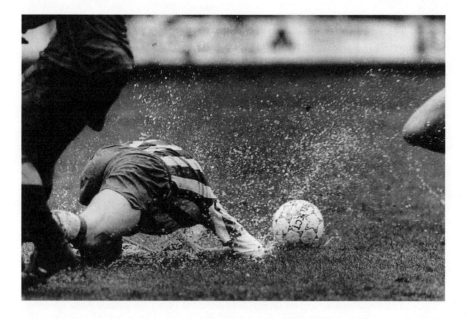

Chapter 9

Bone Mineralization Patterns During Childhood: Relationship to Fractures and Fracture Risk

Cameron J.R. Blimkie and Suzi Kriemler

Introduction

The human skeleton which is comprised of over 200 individual bones serves both as a reservoir for the body's calcium stores (99% of total body calcium), and a framework for the translation of muscle forces into human movement.

Bone strength is dependent largely upon the intrinsic material properties of its inorganic mineral and organic matrix elements. Mineralized matrix (hydroxyapatite) is a major contributor to the material strength of bone tissue, is the primary determinant of bone mineral mass and density, and accounts for about 80%-90% of the variance in bone compressive strength (Genant et al., 1994; Mazess & Wahner, 1988). Other factors besides the material strength and mass density of bone, however, including changes in internal bone microarchitecture and macroscopic changes in bone geometry also contribute substantially to the functional strength or mechanical integrity of the skeleton. This chapter will focus only on development of the inorganic phase of bone, that is the bone mineral element, and its relationship to fracture risk during childhood and adolescence.

Bone tissue is organized structurally into two basic forms; cortical or compact bone, and trabecular or spongy bone. Cortical bone, which forms the outer layer of most bones, and is found mostly in the shafts of the appendicular (limbs) skeleton comprises about 80% of total skeletal mass (Kanis, 1991). Trabecular bone, which is found mostly in the distal portions of long bones, many flat bones, and the vertebral bodies, comprise about 20% of skeletal mass (Kanis, 1991; Parfitt, 1988; Teitelbaum, 1993).

The absolute quantities of cortical and trabecular bone, as well as their proportional distribution vary from bone to bone, within the same bone at different sites and stages of the life-span, between genders, and among individuals and races (Blimkie et al., 1996). Consequently, no one site accurately reflects developmental patterns for purely cortical or trabecular bone types, or is generally representative of mineralization patterns for all other skeletal sites. Emphasis in the following section is placed on developmental patterns of bone mineralization during childhood derived from absorptiometric and computed tomography techniques. Patterns are described for predominantly cortical (the total body and 1/3 distal radius) and trabecular bone (the lumbar spine and femoral neck), with emphasis on gender differences and the influence of puberty.

The technical underpinnings of the absorptiometric and computed tomography techniques for measuring bone mineral in humans, and their relative strengths and limitations have been thoroughly reviewed (Borders et al., 1989; Holbrook et al., 1991; Mazess & Wahner, 1988; Pacifici et al., 1988; Shipp et al., 1988; Tothill, 1989). Both techniques provide highly accurate (within 1-3% of phantom or actual bone specimens) measures of bone mineral in humans. The precision or reproducibility varies slightly from site to site within the skeleton, and ranges between 0.5-2.5% when measured by an experienced technician (Tothill, 1989; Mazess & Wahner, 1988).

Both absorptiometry and computed tomography provide measures of bone mineral mass or content, and a corresponding measure of bone density. There is little controversy over the interpretation of the bone mass or content measure, since this simply reflects the total amount of mineral in a given scan segment. Caution is warranted, however, when interpreting the bone density measure, since this variable is calculated differently for the absorptiometric and computed tomography techniques. With the absorptiometric techniques, the mass equivalent (g or mg) per scanned segment (e.g. for the entire skeleton or the lumbar vertebrae), or the mass equivalent for a standard scan length (e.g. for the radius or femoral neck) is normalized for the projected scan area (segment length x bone width), resulting in areal bone density in units of $g \times cm^{-2}$. With computed tomography, however, the mineral mass is normalized for the bone segment volume, resulting in a true measure of volumetric bone density in units of either $g \times cm^{-3}$ or $mg \times mm^{-3}$.

The aforementioned normalizing approaches have been applied in an attempt to remove the bone size effect (the larger the bone the greater the amount of mineral), thereby facilitating fairer comparisons of mineralization levels across skeletons or segments of skeletons of variable size. The absorptiometric techniques do not account for bone depth or thickness (with the exception of the newest generation DXA scanners which have a lateral scan mode for application at the spine), and unlike computed tomography, are incapable of measuring true bone volume (Blimkie et al., 1996). Failure to correct absorptiometric measures of areal bone density for bone thickness, provides developmental patterns of bone density which systematically underestimate the actual density of smaller compared to larger individuals. This limitation is most problematic during childhood and adolescence because of the dramatic growth-related changes in skeletal size which occur during this period. Absorptiometric measures of areal bone density probably overestimate the true magnitude of change in mineralization which occurs during this period. Computed tomography on the other hand, adequately adjusts for bone size effects by providing equitable comparisons on a per unit volume basis, regardless of age or gender.

Various normalization approaches have been used to overcome the inability of absorptiometry to determine bone volume (Katzman et al., 1991; Kroger et al. 1992; Kroger et al. 1993). With these approaches, bone volume is estimated by multiplying the absorptiometrically determined projected scan area by the thickness or depth of the bone which is also estimated from assumed geometric relationships between scan area and site specific skeletal width or height measurements. Bone mineral content is divided by the estimated volume and the derived measure is bone mineral apparent density (g x cm^{-3}). This measure is similar conceptually to volumetric bone density derived from computed tomography, but is less precise because of the estimated rather than measured bone volume. These differences must be considered when comparing mineralization patterns during the formative growth years, derived from the absorptiometric and computed tomography techniques.

Cortical (predominantly) bone mineralization patterns

Total body bone mineral changes during childhood

Total body bone mineral content (BMC) and areal bone density (BMD) increase significantly between early childhood and late adolescence (Figure 1 page 114) in both genders (Faulkner et al., 1993; Geusens et al., 1991; Lu et al., 1994; Rico et al., 1992). The rates of gain in BMC and BMD are similar for both genders (Lu et al., 1994), and there is no evidence of a significant gender difference for these measures prior to adolescence; values appear to be higher, however, for males during adolescence (Faulkner et al., 1993; Geusens et al., 1991; Lu et al., 1994). Peak BMC and areal BMD are not achieved until the last few years of the second decade or during the 3rd decade in both genders (Faulkner et al., 1993; Geusens et al., 1991; Lu et al., 1994).

In the only study to date which has attempted to correct absorptiometric measures for bone size (Katzman et al., 1991), there was no change in volumetric total body BMD (bone mineral apparent density) in females between 9 and 20 years of age. This suggests that the large increases in uncorrected areal BMD during childhood reported in other studies is an overestimate of changes in true volumetric mineral density during the childhood period.

Changes during puberty

Total body areal BMC and BMD increase more rapidly (approximate increases of 75-100% and 15-25%, respectively) during the circumpubertal years (10-15 years of age) than at times prior to or following this period (Figure 2 page 115) for both sexes (Faulkner et al., 1993a; Geusens et al., 1991; Katzman et al., 1991; Lu et al., 1994). In healthy non-athletic adolescent females, neither total body BMC or BMD are correlated with age of onset of menarche (Lu et al., 1994; Rice et al., 1993). Recently, however, a significant negative correlation has been reported between age at menarche and total body BMD in competitive female gymnasts (Robinson et al., 1995). In contrast, BMD, appears to be significantly positively correlated with years post menarche, but only during the first two years following the onset of menstruation (Lu et al., 1994).

Figure 1: Changes in total body BMC and areal BMD during childhood. Adapted from Geusens et al., 1991 (panel a), and Lu et al., 1994 (panel b).

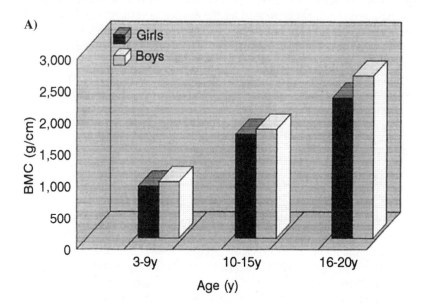

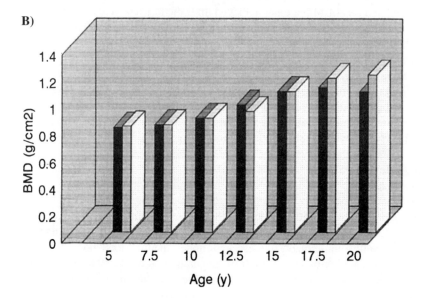

Figure 2: Changes in total body BMC and areal BMD during the circum-pubertal years. Adapted from Faulkner et al., 1993.

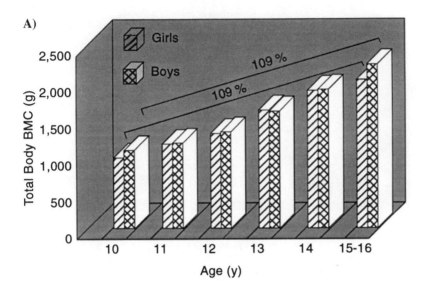

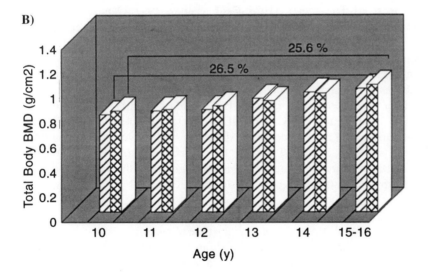

Distal radial bone mineral changes during childhood

Radial BMC and areal BMD (Figure 3 page 116) increase progressively and sub-stantially with increasing age from early childhood to late adolescence for both genders (Bell et al., 1991; Geusens et al., 1991; Hagino et al., 1990; Li et al., 1989; Rubin et al., 1993; Sugimoto et al., 1994). BMC and BMD increase at a steady rate

Figure 3: Changes in radial cortical (1/3 distal radial) areal BMD during childhood. Adapted from Hagino et al., 1990.

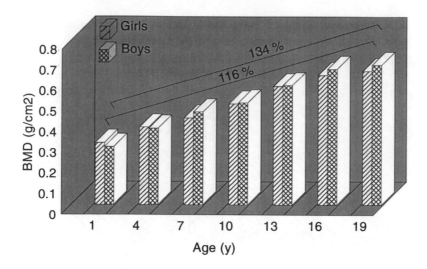

during the prepubertal years and accelerate in both genders during the circumpubertal years (Christiansen et al., 1975; Geusens et al., 1991; Gunnes et al., 1994; Katzman et al., 1991; Krabbe et al., 1979; Krabbe et al., 1984 a,b; Riss et al., 1985; Rubin et al., 1993). There is little if any gender difference in BMC or BMD during the prepubertal and early pubertal years, values are higher generally for boys beginning in late adolescence, and the difference becomes even more accentuated with increasing age into early adulthood (Christiansen et al., 1975; Geusens et al., 1991; Hagino et al., 1990; Krabbe et al., 1979; Rubin et al., 1993; Sugimoto et al., 1994). For females, radial BMC and BMD appear to reach peak levels during the fourth or early part of the fifth decades (Aloia et al., 1985; Falch & Sandvik, 1990; Geusens et al., 1986; Mazess & Barden, 1991; Prentice et al., 1991). Peak radial BMC and BMD for males occurs between the latter part of the third or early part of the fourth decades (Geusens et al., 1986; Hannan et al., 1992).

Changes during puberty
Both radial BMC and BMD accelerate at the time of puberty in both sexes (Figure 4). About 50% of the total change in BMC from childhood to adulthood and more than half of the change in BMD (50% and 75 %, respectively for girls and boys) occurs during the pubertal years (Geusens et al., 1991). The absolute magnitude of the increase in both BMC and BMD appear to be greater for males than females during the pubertal years, and values for both measures continue to increase between adolescence and adulthood for males, whereas females demonstrate smaller gains or a plateau during the same period (Christiansen et al., 1975; Geusens et al., 1991; Gunnes et al., 1994; Hagino et al., 1990; Krabbe et al., 1979; Sugimoto et al., 1994). BMD changes slowly and appears to plateau for females

Figure 4: Changes in radial cortical (1/3 distal radius) BMC and areal BMD during the circumpubertal years. Adapted from Geusens et al., 1991.

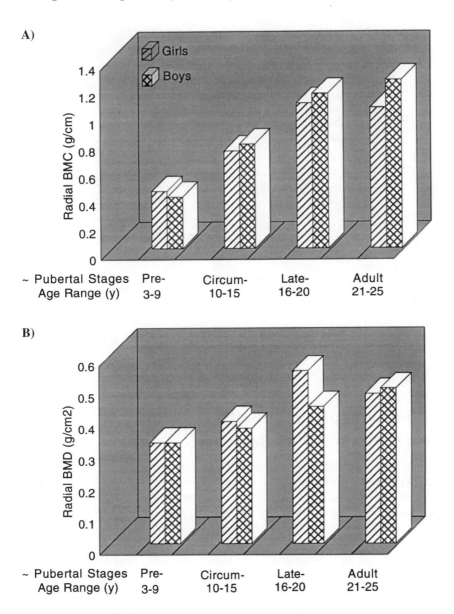

during the latter stages of puberty (Geusens et al., 1991; Katzman et al., 1991; Matkovic et al., 1990; Rubin et al., 1993), whereas it continues to increase for males from late puberty until early adulthood (Geusens et al., 1991; Rubin et al., 1993). One study failed to demonstrate an acceleration in radial BMD for females

Figure 5: Changes in radial cortical areal BMD in relation to menarche. Adapted from Gunnes, 1994.

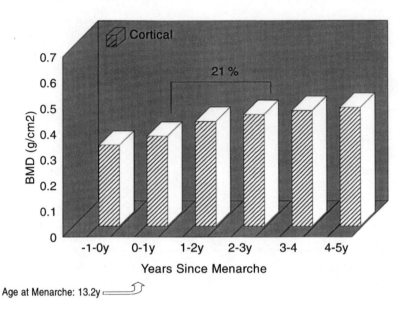

during the pubertal years (Rubin et al., 1993), whereas another (Figue 5) reported that the largest pubertal gains in BMD occurred during the first 2 years following the onset of menarche (Gunnes, 1994).

Trabecular (predominantly) bone mineralization patterns

Femoral neck bone mineral changes during childhood

There is only one published report of actual changes in femoral neck BMC with age during childhood (Katzman et al., 1991). In this study BMC increased in a curvilinear fashion by about 80-90% with increasing age for females between 9 and 21 years of age. Femoral neck BMC, however, has been reported to be significantly positively correlated with age in both sexes between 3 and 18 years (Kroger et al., 1992; Thomas et al., 1991). There are no reports of a significant sex difference in femoral neck BMC during childhood. Femoral neck areal BMD increases significantly and substantially (Figure 6a) between early childhood and the mid-teens for females, and the late teens for males (Kroger et al., 1993; Lu et al., 1994; Thomas et al., 1991). There is considerable variability in reported annual rates of increase in femoral neck areal BMD, with the range of values being slightly higher in males than in females (Kroger et al., 1993; Thomas et al., 1991). Gender differences in femoral neck areal BMD during the prepubertal and early pubertal years remain equivocal (Bonjour et al., 1991; Grimston et al., 1992; Kroger et al.,

1992; Kroger et al., 1993; Lu et al., 1994; Miller et al., 1991; Thomas et al., 1991). Males consistently have higher femoral neck BMD than females during late adolescence; the difference in some studies is quite small and not significant (Bonjour et al., 1991; Grimston et al., 1992; Kroger et al., 1992; Thomas et al., 1991), whereas others report larger differences which were not tested statistically (Kroger et al., 1993; Lu et al., 1994). In females, femoral neck BMC and BMD both appear to peak between the latter part of the second and the fourth decades (Cazes et al., 1994; Latinen et al., 1991; Mazess & Barden, 1991; Rodin et al., 1990). Peak values for males occur during early adulthood (Blimkie et al., 1996; Blunt et al., 1994).

Figure 6: Changes in femoral neck areal BMD and apparent BMD (BMAD) during childhood. Adapted from Kroger et al., 1993.

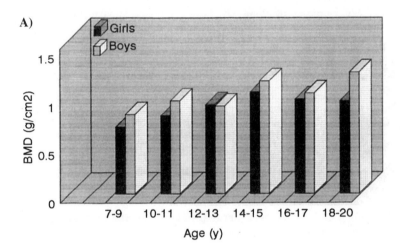

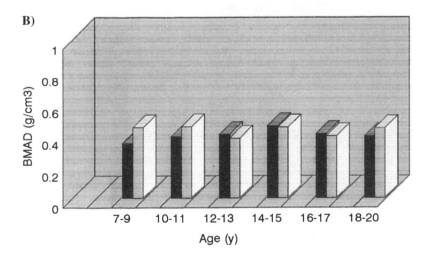

A few studies have reported developmental changes in femoral neck BMD corrected for changes in bone size. In one study (Kroger et al., 1992), volumetric BMD did not change appreciably for females or males between 7 and 19 years of age (Figure 6b). There is apparently no correlation between age and volumetric BMD, and no significant sex difference in volumetric BMD at comparable ages (Katzman et al., 1991; Kroger et al., 1992; Kroger et al., 1993). The largest increases in volumetric BMD occured between 12-15 years and 14-17 years of age for males and females (Kroger et al., 1993). These observations suggest that the aforementioned age-related increases and gender differences in femoral neck areal BMD were due primarily to bone expansion with growth, and to sexual dimorphism in bone size during childhood.

Changes during puberty
Femoral neck BMC increased by about 55% between 10 and 16 years of age in females (Katzman et al., 1991). Femoral neck areal BMD increases with advancing level of sexual maturity in both genders (Figure 7), during the circumpubertal years (Bonjour et al., 1991; Grimston et al., 1992; Henderson, 1991; Katzman et al., 1991; Kroger et al., 1992; Miller et al., 1991; Slemenda et al., 1994; Theintz et al., 1992; Thomas et al., 1991), accounting for between 25-35% of the overall increase in BMD during the entire growth period (Bonjour et al., 1991; Grimston et al, 1992; Kroger et al., 1993; Lu et al., 1994; Theintz et al., 1992). In one study (Kroger et al., 1993), the peak rate of change in femoral neck BMD for females occurred during the year prior to menarche; the rate decreased substantially with increasing age and level of sexual maturity following the onset of menarche. One study (Lu et al., 1994) failed to find any relationship between age of onset of

Figure 7: Changes in femoral neck areal BMD during the circumpubertal years. Adapted from Bonjour et al., 1991.

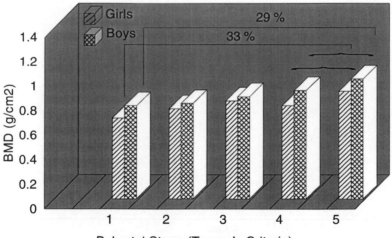

menarche and femoral neck BMD in healthy non-athletic females, whereas another recent study (Robinson et al., 1995) found a negative correlation in competitive female gymnasts.

Vertebral bone mineral changes during childhood

Lumbar spine BMC and areal BMD increase with increasing age (Figure 8 page 122) from early childhood until the mid-teens for females, and the late teens for males (Bell et al., 1991; Bonjour et al., 1991; Del Rio et al., 1994; DeSchepper et al., 1991; Geusens et al., 1991; Glastre et al., 1990; Henderson & Hayes, 1994; Katzman et al., 1991; Kroger et al., 1992; Kroger et al., 1993; Lu et al., 1994; McCormick et al., 1991; Ponder et al., 1990; Rubin et al., 1993; Southard et al., 1991; Thomas et al., 1991). Both BMC and areal BMD are highly positively correlated with age throughout childhood for males, but only up to mid-puberty for females (Bell et al., 1991; del Rio et. al., 1994; DeSchepper et al., 1991; Geusens et al., 1991; Glastre et al., 1990; Henderson & Hayes, 1994; Katzman et al., 1991; Kroger et al., 1992; Lu et al., 1994; McCormick et al., 1991; Ponder et al., 1990; Rubin et al., 1993; Southard et al., 1991; Thomas et al., 1991). Neither BMC or areal BMD are correlated with age in females between 14 and 18 years of age (Bonjour et al., 1991; del Rio et al., 1994; DeSchepper et al., 1991; Guesens et al., 1991; Katzman et al., 1991; Lu et al., 1994; Rice et al., 1993; White et al., 1992). There appears to be little if any gender difference in BMC or BMD during the prepubertal years, but females tend to have slightly or significantly higher values than males during the initial years of the circumpubertal period (9-15 years of age), and somewhat lower values during the later years of adolescence (Bonjour et al., 1991; del Rio et al., 1994; DeSchepper et al., 1991; Geusens et al., 1991; Glastre et al., 1990; Grimston et al., 1992; Henderson & Hayes, 1994; Kroger et al., 1993; Lu et al., 1994; McCormick et al., 1991; Miller et al., 1991; Rubin et al., 1993). The maximal rate of gain for BMC and areal BMD occurs in both sexes between 1 and 3 years of age (del Rio et al., 1994). In females, lumbar spine BMC and BMD both appear to peak sometime after adolescence, during either the third or fourth decades (Blimkie et al., 1996; Casez et al., 1994; Mazess & Barden, 1991; Rico et al., 1991). Peak BMC and BMD for males appears to occur during the third decade (Cann et al., 1985; Compston et al., 1988; Geusens et al., 1986; Hagiwara et al., 1989).

Lumbar spine apparent volumetric density (Figure 9 page 123) increases until the mid-teens for females and the late teens for males (Katzman et al., 1991; Kroger et al. 1992; Kroger et al., 1993). Females have slightly higher apparent volumetric density than males during most of childhood, and this difference is maintained even during adolescence (Kroger et al., 1992; Kroger et al., 1993). Apparent density increases by 20-30% between 7 and 18 years of age, with about similar gains in both genders (Katzman et al., 1991; Kroger et al., 1992; Kroger et al., 1993).

Changes in true volumetric density of the lumbar spine during childhood have also been determined by computed tomography. Based on limited data, it appears (Figure 10 page 124) that true volumetric density of the lumbar spine trabecular bone

Figure 8: Changes in lumbar spine BMC and areal BMD during childhood. Adapted from del Rio et al., 1994.

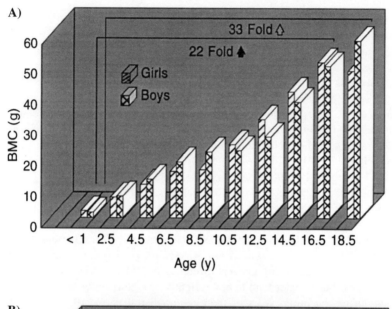

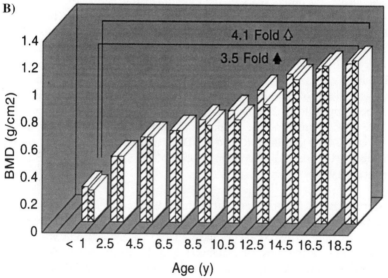

compartment increases only slightly and insignificantly in both sexes during the pre- and early-pubertal years up to about 11.5 and 14 years of age in females and males, respectively (Gilsanz et al., 1988a,b; Gilsanz et al., 1991; Gilsanz et al., 1994). Lumbar spine volumetric density increases by less than 25% in white males

Figure 9: Changes in lumbar spine apparent BMD during childhood. Adapted from Kroger et al., 1993.

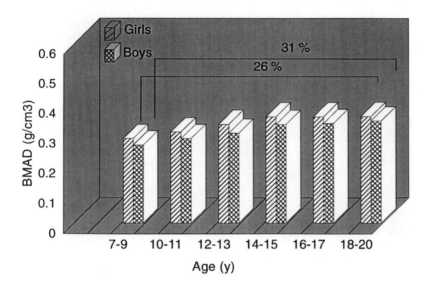

and females from early childhood to adulthood (Gilsanz et al., 1988a,b,; Gilsanz et al., 1991). There is no apparent gender difference in lumbar spine volumetric density at any age or stage of sexual maturity during childhood (Gilsanz et al., 1988b; Gilsanz et al., 1994b).

Changes during puberty

Lumbar spine BMC increases with advancing level of sexual maturity in both sexes (Bonjour et al., 1991; DeSchepper et al., 1991; Katzman et al., 1991; Miller et al., 1991), with proportionately larger increases in females compared to males during the circumpubertal years (del Rio et al., 1994; DeSchepper et al., 1991; Geusens et al., 1991; Gordon et al., 1991). Lumbar spine areal BMD increases dramatically between 10-15 years of age for females and 13-17 years of age for males (Figure 8b page 122), and increases with level of sexual maturity in both genders; density is highest in the most sexually mature individuals, and is similar between genders at comparable levels of maturity (Bonjour et al., 1991; Del Rio et al., 1994; DeSchepper et al., 1991; Grimston et al., 1992; Katzman et al., 1991; Kroger et al., 1993; Rubin et al., 1993; Sentipal et al., 1991; Slemenda et al., 1994; Southard et al. 1991).

There is no clear gender difference in the magnitude of change that occurs in lumbar areal BMD during puberty (Bonjour et al. 1991; del Rio et al., 1994; Gordon et al., 1991; Grimston et al., 1992; Kroger et al., 1993; McCormick et al., 1991; Rubin et al., 1993). The largest increase in BMD appears to occur in both genders between Tanner pubertal stages 3 and 5 (commencing at about 13.5 y for girls), and there is no significant gender difference in the maximal rate of gain in

Figure 10: Changes in volumetric vertebral BMD during childhood. Adapted from Gilsanz et al., 1988.

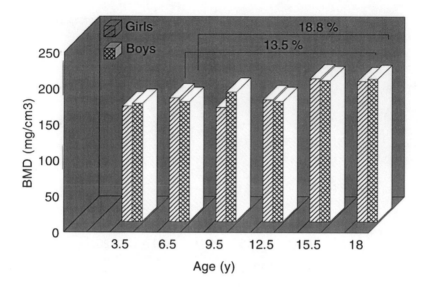

BMD during this period (Bonjour et al., 1991; del Rio et al., 1994; DeSchepper et al., 1991; Glastre et al., 1990; Grimston et al., 1992; Kroger et al., 1993; Rubin et al., 1993; Southard et al., 1991; Theintz et al., 1992). Two studies (Lu et al., 1994; Rice et al., 1993) failed to find a significant correlation between age at onset of menarche and BMD in healthy non-athletic females, whereas a recent study (Robinson et al., 1995) reported a negative correlation in young competitive gymnasts. The largest increase in areal BMD during the circumpubertal period (Figure 11) appears to occur in females between pubertal stages 4 and 5 which corresponds to the first few years following the onset of menses (Bonjour et al., 1991; Katzman et al., 1991; Theintz et al., 1992). In boys, the greatest increase occurs between pubertal stages 3 and 4.

Apparent volumetric BMD (determined by absorptiometry) experiences its largest increase between 11-13 years of age for females and 13-17 years of age for males (Kroger et al., 1993). In females, the maximal rate of gain in apparent volumetric BMD is coincident with the onset of menarche (Kroger et al., 1993). The maximal rate of change and the average annual rate of change in apparent volumetric BMD are slightly higher in females compared to males, and lower than changes in areal BMD (Kroger et al., 1993). The latter observation suggests that absorptiometrically determined areal BMD measures probably overestimate true volumetric changes in BMD during this period of rapid growth.

Lumbar spine volumetric BMD determined by computed tomography increases rather dramatically in both sexes (Figure 12) during the pubertal years, especially from mid-puberty to post puberty (puberty stages III to V), and plateaus at about

Figure 11: Changes in lumbar spine areal BMD during the circumpubertal years. Adapted from Bonjour et al., 1991.

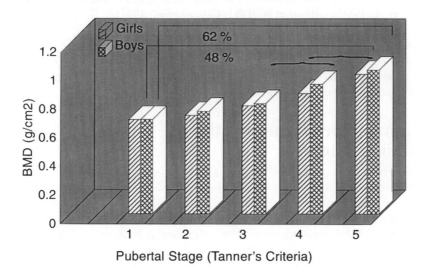

Figure 12: Changes in lumbar spine volumetric BMD during the circumpubertal years. Adapted from Gilsanz et al., 1988.

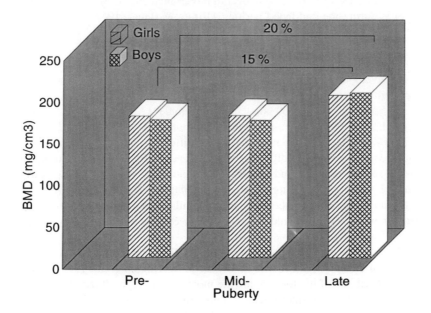

the same level in both genders during late adolescence (Gilsanz et al., 1988a,b; Gilsanz et al., 1991; Gilsanz et al., 1994b). About 80-90% of the total gain in volumetric BMD during childhood occurs in whites between mid- and post-puberty (Gilsanz et al., 1988b; Gilsanz et al., 1991; Gilsanz et al., 1994).

Bone mineral content and density are important determinants of bone strength and skeletal susceptibility to fracture. The following section describes the association between developmental changes in bone mineral status and fracture incidence and risk during childhood and adolescence.

Epidemiologic characteristics of childhood fractures

Fracture incidence increases progressively with age in both sexes during the prepubertal years, peaks at extremely high levels during the circumpubertal years, and then declines progressively with age (Figure 13) throughout adolescence and into early adulthood (Alffram & Bauer, 1962; Bailey et al., 1989; Blimkie et al., 1993; Hagino et al., 1990; Kleerekoper et al., 1981; Kramhoft & Bodtker, 1988; Landin, 1983). Compared to girls, boys have the same or slightly higher fracture incidence during the prepubertal and later years of adolescence (Alffram & Bauer, 1962; Bailey et al., 1989; Hagino et al., 1990; Kramhoft & Bodtker, 1988). Several (Bailey et al., 1989; Hagino et al., 1990; Landin, 1983), but not all studies (Alffram & Bauer, 1962; Kramhoft & Bodtker, 1988), however, indicate an approximate two fold higher fracture incidence in boys compared to girls during the circumpubertal years. Generally, however, there is an overall higher incidence of fractures in boys than in girls during the childhood period (Alffram & Bauer, 1962; Kramhoft & Bodtker, 1988; Landin, 1983).

Absolute fracture incidence varies considerably across studies at given ages and stages of development during childhood: peak fracture incidence during the circumpubertal years ranges between 12 and 500 per 10,000 population for males, and 5 and 250 per 10,000 population for females (Alffram & Bauer, 1962; Bailey et al., 1989; Hagino et al., 1990; Kramhoft & Bodtker, 1988; Landin, 1983). This variability may be attributed to the different approaches used in calculating fracture incidence, to differences in the types of fractures included in the analysis, to secular changes, and to socio-economic differences (including nutritional and physical activity histories) among populations. Despite this variability, peak rates during the circumpubertal years are similar to population specific rates reported for women in their mid-fifties (Alffram & Bauer, 1962; Bailey et al., 1989).

Most fractures during childhood occur at the relatively undermineralized metaphyseal region of long bones (Davis & Green, 1976; Hagino et al., 1990). Fractures to the distal end of the forearm are the most common type (Figure 14a page 128), followed by forearm shaft fractures; approximately 80% of all lifetime forearm shaft fractures occur during childhood (Alffram & Bauer, 1962; Landin, 1983). Fractures to the physes (growth plate) comprise about 10% of all fractures

Figure 13: Fracture incidence in Swedish and Canadian populations. Adapted from Alffram & Bauer, 1962 (panel a) and Bailey et al., 1989 (panel b).

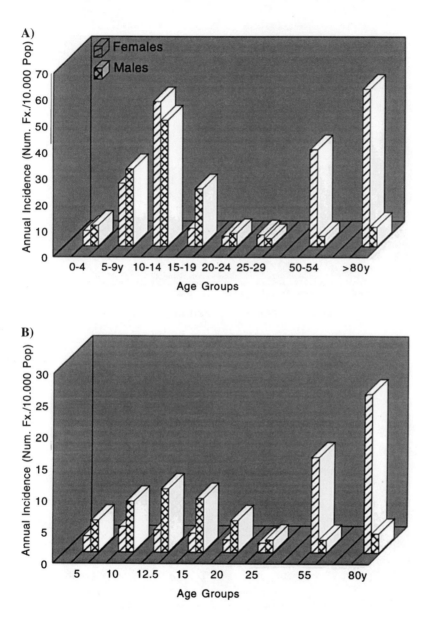

Figure 14: Fracture characteristics during childhood. Adapted from Alffram & Bauer, 1962.

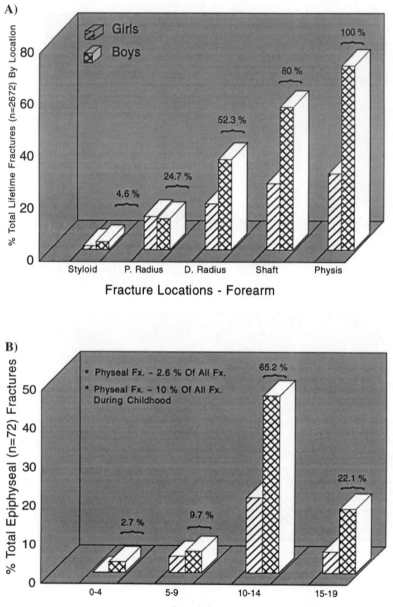

during the childhood period, but only about 2% of all radial fractures throughout the lifespan (Alffram & Bauer, 1962; Kramhoft & Bodtker, 1988). Physeal fracture incidence (Figure 14b) increases dramatically between 10 and 15 years of age, and there are more physeal fractures in boys than girls (Alffram & Bauer, 1962; Landin, 1983) during this period.

Unlike osteoporotic fractures, fractures during childhood are often associated with some degree of trauma (Alffram & Bauer, 1962; Blimkie et al., 1993; Landin, 1983; Melton, 1988). The majority of fractures throughout childhood are associated with slight to moderate trauma (Alffram & Bauer, 1962; Landin, 1983). Although the number of fractures associated with severe trauma increases slightly during the circumpubertal years in both sexes, there is nevertheless a reduction in the ratio of moderate/severe trauma associated with fractures during this period compared to the previous and following decades (Alffram & Bauer, 1962). This latter observation suggests an increase in bone fragility and increased susceptibility to fracture during this period.

Influence of growth on bone mineralization
The peak fracture incidence during childhood occurs coincidentally with the growth spurt in stature in both boys and girls (Bailey et al., 1989; Blimkie et al., 1993; Kleerekoper et al., 1981). Paradoxically, this is also the period of largest lifetime gains in bone mineral mass and density (see previous section). These observations suggest an uncoupling of the normal relationship between bone mineralization and fracture risk during the circumpubertal period.

An alternative hypothesis, however, proposes a developmental lag between linear growth (length and width) of the skeleton and bone mineralization during this period. A relative lag in the rate of bone mineralization in relation to linear growth would temporarily render bones more fragile, predisposing to increased fracture risk and rates. A recent study reported a 6 month lag in the timing of peak growth rates for metacarpal cortical thickness relative to the timing of peak growth rates for stature and metacarpal length (Blimkie et al., 1993) in adolescent boys. This observation lends support to the concept that a developmental delay in bone mineralization relative to linear skeletal growth may contribute to the increased fracture rates observed during this period.

The increased fracture incidence during the growth spurt has also been postulated to be due to increased intra-cortical bone turnover and cortical porosity during this stage of development (Parfitt, 1994). Increased intra-cortical bone turnover would provide additional calcium in support of the rapid growth in bone length and width at the metaphysis, but at the expense of temporarily incomplete or delayed cortical bone mineralization and increased bone fragility at the diaphysis. The peak fracture incidence for the distal radius occurs coincidentally with the nadir in the ratio of metaphyseal to diaphyseal BMD in both sexes during the circumpubertal years (Hagino et al., 1990). This observation supports Parfitt's (1994) postulation, and suggests that normal growth dynamics may place children at increased risk for fracture during the circumpubertal years. No study to date, however, has prospectively assessed the inter-relationship between rates of bone mineralization, bone growth (length and width), and skeletal fractures during this stage of the lifespan.

Relationship between bone mineral status and fractures
The relationship between fracture susceptibility and bone mineral status in children with pathological conditions is fairly well established. There is an unequivocal positive association between reduced bone mineral mass and density and increased fracture incidence in children with idiopathic juvenile osteoporosis (Smith, 1980), osteogenesis imperfecta and rheumatoid arthritis (Landin, 1983) and adolescent females with menstrual dysfunction (Figure 15a) or eating disorders (Marcus et al., 1985; Warren et al., 1991).

The association between fracture susceptibility and bone mineral status in otherwise healthy children, however, is somewhat more equivocal. Several studies have reported no significant difference (Figure 15b) in bone mineral status between children with and without fractures (Blimkie et al., 1993; Cook et al., 1987; De-Schepper et al., 1991), whereas others have reported lower than normal (age

Figure 15: Relationship between fracture incidence and bone mineral status during childhood. Adapted from Warren et al., 1991 (panel a), Cook et al., 1987 (panel b), and Chan et al., 1984 (panel c).

Relationship Between Bone Mineral Status And Fractures

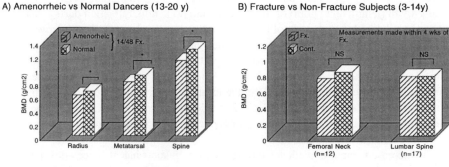

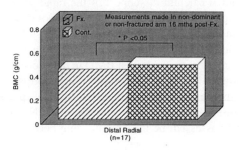

matched controls) bone mineral content and density (Figure 15c) in pediatric fracture populations (Chan et al., 1984; Landin & Nilsson, 1983). These studies are
usually conducted on the contralateral non-fractured limb after the fracture has occured, generally provide no information about pre-existing bone mineral status,
rarely indicate the location of bone mineral measurements relative to the fracture
site, and fail to control for other factors which could influence susceptibility to
fracture including nutritional and physical activity status, and severity of the
initiating trauma at the time of fracture. It appears from these studies that absolute
reductions in BMC and BMD are sufficient, but not necessary antecedents to increased fracture incidence during childhood. There are no prospective studies to
our knowledge of the relationship between fracture incidence and bone mineral
status during childhood which have controlled for these influences. Future studies
should incorporate bone mineral measurements at the most common fracture sites
for children (e.g. shaft, diaphysis and metaphysis of long bones), while controlling
for these extraneous factors.

Relationship between physical activity and fractures
The increased incidence of fractures during the circumpubertal years is generally
attributed to concurrent increases in level of physical activity. As pointed out by
Parfitt (1994), however, it is unlikely that activity levels during the circumpubertal
years differ sufficiently from the years immediately before and following the
growth spurt to account for the increased fracture incidence. Physical activity
level (time per week) in one study of adolescent Belgian boys (Blimkie et al.,
1993) peaked about 2-3 years later than the peak fracture incidence (Figure 16),
and participation rates in physical activity by Canadian Boys remained high and

**Figure 16: Relationship between fracture frequency and physical activity pat-
terns in Belgian boys. Adapted from Blimkie et al., 1993.**

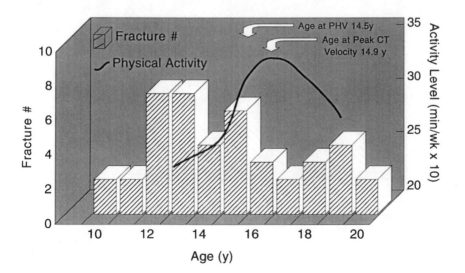

Figure 17: Activities associated with fractures during childhood. Adapted from Landin, 1983 (panel a), and Blimkie et al., 1993 (panel b).

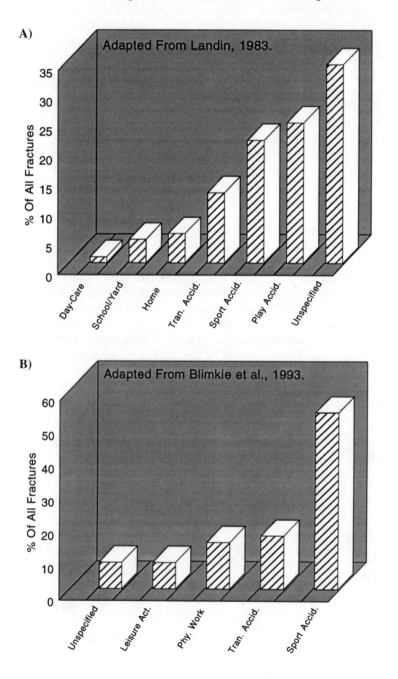

unchanged from the circumpubertal years during late adolescence (Canada Fitness Survey, 1983), when fracture incidence of the distal radius was declining toward its nadir (Bailey et al., 1989). Activity patterns are more closely matched with radial fracture incidence for girls, with peak participation rates and fracture incidence occuring during early puberty, and then both declining toward their nadir in early adulthood (Bailey et al., 1989; Canada Fitness Survey, 1983).

It is clear from epidemiological studies, though, that a large proportion of fractures (Figure 17) during childhood and adolescence are associated with acute trauma incurred while participating in sport or general physical activity (Alffram & Bauer, 1962; Blimkie et al., 1993; Kramhoft & Bodtker, 1988; Landin, 1983). Other factors however, besides increased participation rates and time spent in physical activity, including for example, the intensity of participation, the level of aggressiveness of participation, and the effect of increased body mass on impact forces, cannot be discounted as contributing factors to the increased fracture incidence in the transition from the prepubertal to circumpubertal years in both sexes.

Little attention has been given to the economic costs associated with the increased fracture incidence during the circumpubertal years, and to the effects of ensuing restricted activity on peak BMD and subsequent risk of fracture in old age. Achieving and maintaining the highest possible BMC and BMD appears a necessary, but not necessarily sufficient prerequisite to insure adequate bone strength to protect against risk of fractures during childhood. Fracture risk during childhood may be minimized by ensuring adequate levels of safe physical activity, a proper diet, and a supportive endocrine environment to ensure optimal bone mineral development.

Acknowledgements

The authors thank Dr. Colin Webber, and Dr. J.D. (Rick) Adachi for their continued collaboration and support. Appreciation is also extended to the Ontario Ministry of Tourism and Recreation, Fitness Branch, and Sport Canada for their financial support of the authors' work in this area. Authors' mailing addresses: [1] Department of Kinesiology, McMaster University, Hamilton, Ontario, Canada, and [2] Children's Exercise and Nutrition Center, Chedoke Hospital, Hamilton, Canada.

References

Alffram, P.-E., and G.C.H. Bauer (1962). Epidemiology of fractures of the forearm. J. Bone Joint Surg. 44-A: 105-114.

Bailey, D.A., J.H. Wedge, R.G. McCulloch, A.D. Martin, and S.C. Bernhardson (1989). Epidemiology of fractures of the distal end of the radius in children as associated with growth. J. Bone Joint Surg. 71-A: 1225-1231.

Bell, N.H., J. Shary, J. Stevens, M. Garza, L. Gordon, and J. Edwards (1991). Demonstration that bone mass is greater in black than in white children. J. Bone Miner. Res. 6: 719-723.

Blimkie, C.J.R., J. Lefevre, G.P. Beunen, R. Renson, J. Dequeker, and P. Van Damme (1993). Fractures, physical activity, and growth velocity in adolescent Belgian boys. Med. Sci. Sports Exerc. 25: 801-808.

Blimkie, C.J.R., P.D. Chilibeck, and K.S. Davison (1996). Bone mineralization patterns: reproductive endocrine, nutrition, and physical activity influences during the lifespan. In: Perspectives In Exercise and Sports Medicine. Vol. 9. Exercise and the Female – A Lifespan Perspective. O. Bar-Or, D. Lamb, and P. Clarkson (eds.). Cooper Publishing Group.

Blunt, B.A., M.R. Klauber, E.L. Barrett-Connor, and S.L. Edelstein (1994). Sex differences in bone mineral density in 1653 men and women in the sixth through tenth decades of life: The Rancho Bernardo study. J. Bone Miner. Res. 9: 1333-1338.

Bonjour, J.-P., G. Theintz, B. Buchs, D. Slosman, and R. Rizzoli (1991). Critical years and stages of puberty for spinal and femoral bone mass accumulation during adolescence. J. Clin. Endocrinol. Metab. 73: 555-563.

Borders, J., E. Kerr, D.J. Sartoris, J.A. Stein, E. Ramos, A.A. Moscona, and D. Resnick (1989). Quantitative dual-energy radiographic absorptiometry of the lumbar spine: In vivo comparison with dual-photon absorptiometry. Radiology 170: 129-131.

Canada Fitness Survey (1983). Canadian Youth and Physical Activity. Ottawa: Fitness and Amateur Sport.

Cann, C.E., H.K. Genant, F.O. Kolb, and B. Ettinger (1985). Quantitative computed tomography for prediction of vertebral fracture risk. Bone 6: 1-7.

Casez, J.-P., A. Troendle, K. Lippuner, and P. Jaeger (1994). Bone mineral density at distal tibia using dual-energy x-ray absorptiometry in normal women and in patients with vertebral osteoporosis or primary hyperparathyroidism. J. Bone Miner. Res. 9: 1851-1857.

Chan, G., M. Hess, J. Hollis, and L. Book (1984). Bone mineral status in childhood accidental fractures. Am. J. Dis. Child. 138: 569-570.

Christiansen, C., P. Rodbro, and C. T. Nielsen (1975). Bone mineral content and estimated total body calcium in normal children and adolescents. Scand. J. Clin. Lab. Invest. 35: 507-510.

Compston, J.E., W.D. Evans, E.O. Crawley, and C. Evans (1988). Bone mineral content in normal UK subjects. Br. J. Radiol. 61: 631-636.

Cook, S.D., A.F. Harding, E.L. Morgan, H.J. Doucet, J.T. Bennett, M.O'Brien, and K.A. Thomas (1987). Association of bone mineral density and pediatric fractures. J. Pediatr. Orthop. 7: 424-427.

Davis, D.R., and D.P. Green (1976). Forearm fractures in children. Pitfalls and complications. Clin. Orthop. 120: 172-184.

del Rio, L., A. Carrascosa, F. Pons, M. Gusinye, D. Yeste, and F.M. Domenech (1994). Bone mineral density of the lumbar spine in white mediterranean Spanish children and adolescents: Changes related to age, sex, and puberty. Pediatr. Res. 35: 362-366.

DeSchepper, J., M.P. Derde, M. Van Den Broeck, A. Piepsz, and M.H. Jonckheer (1991). Normative data for lumbar spine bone mineral content in children: Influence of age, height, weight, and pubertal stage. J. Nucl. Med. 32: 216-220.

Faulkner, R.A., D.A. Bailey, D.T. Drinkwater, A.A. Wilkinson, C.S. Houston, and H.A. McKay (1993). Regional and total body bone mineral content, bone mineral density, and total body tissue composition in children 8-16 years of age. Calcif. Tissue Int. 53: 7-12, 1993.

Genant, H.K., C.-C. Gluer, and J.C. Lotz (1994). Gender differences in bone density, skeletal geometry, and fracture biomechanics. Radiology 190: 636-640.

Geusens, P., F. Cantatore, J. Nijs, W. Proesmans, F. Emma, and J. Dequeker (1991). Heterogeneity of growth of bone in children at the spine, radius and total skeleton. Growth Dev. Aging 55: 249-256.

Geusens, P., J. Dequeker, A. Verstraeten, and J. Nijs (1986). Age-, sex-, and menopause-related changes of vertebral and peripheral bone: Population study using dual and single photon absorptiometry and radiogrammetry. J. Nuc. Med. 27: 1540-1549.

Gilsanz, V., M.I. Boechat, T.F. Roe, M.L. Loro, J.W. Sayre, and W.G. Goodman (1994). Gender differences in vertebral body sizes in children and adolescents. Radiology 190: 673-677.

Gilsanz, V., D.T. Gibbens, M. Carlson, M.I. Boechat, C.E. Cann, and E.E. Schulz (1988a). Peak trabecular vertebral density: a comparison of adolescent and adult females. Calcif. Tissue Int. 43: 260-262.

Gilsanz, V., D.T. Gibbens, T.F. Roe, M. Carlson, M.O. Senac, M.I. Boechat, H.K. Huang, E.E. Schulz, C.R. Libanati, and C.C. Cann (1988b). Vertebral bone density in children: effect of puberty. Radiol. 166: 847-850.

Gilsanz, V., T.F. Roe, S. Mora, G. Costin, and W.G. Goodman (1991). Changes in vertebral bone density in black and white girls during childhood and puberty. N. Engl. J. Med. 325: 1597-1600.

Glastre, C., P. Braillon, L. David, P. Cochat, P.J. Meunier, and P.D. Delmas (1990). Measurement of bone mineral content of the lumbar spine by dual energy x-ray absorptiometry in normal children: correlations with growth parameters. J. Clin. Endocrinol. Metab. 70: 1330-1333.

Gordon, C.L., J.M. Halton, S.A. Atkinson, and C.E. Webber (1991). The contributions of growth and puberty to peak bone mass. Growth Develop. Ageing 55: 257-262.

Grimston, S.K., K. Morrison, J.A. Harder, and D.A. Hanley (1992). Bone mineral density during puberty in western Canadian children. Bone Miner. 19: 85-96.

Gunnes, M. (1994). Bone mineral density in the cortical and trabecular distal forearm in healthy children and adolescents. Acta. Paediatr. 83: 463-467.

Hagino, H., K. Yamamoto, R. Teshima, H. Kishimoto, and T. Nakamura (1990). Fracture incidence and bone mineral density of the distal radius in Japanese children. Arch. Orthop. Trauma Surg. 109: 262-264.

Hagiwara, S., T. Miki, Y. Nishizawa, H. Ochi, Y., Onoyama, and H. Morii (1989). Quantification of bone mineral content using dual-photon absorptiometry in a normal Japanese population. J. Bone Miner. Res. 4: 217-222.

Hannan, M.T., D.T. Felson, and J.J. Anderson (1992). Bone mineral density in elderly women: results from the Framingham Osteoporosis study. J. Bone Miner. Res. 7: 547-553.

Henderson, R.C. (1991). Assessment of bone mineral content in children. J. Pediatr. Orthop. 11: 314-317.

Henderson, R.C., and P.R.L. Hayes (1994). Bone mineralization in children and adolescents with a milk allergy. Bone Miner. 27: 1-12.

Holbrook, T.L., E. Barnett-Connor, M. Klauber, and D. Sartoris (1991). A population based comparison of quantitative dual-energy absorptiometry with dual-photon absorptiometry of the spine and legs. Calcif. Tissue Int. 49: 305-307.

Kanis, J.A. (1991). Pathophysiology and histopathology. In: J.A. Kanis (ed.) Pathophysiology and Treatment of Paget's Disease of Bone. London: Martin Dunitz, pp. 12-40.

Katzman, D.K., L.K. Bachrach, D.R. Carter, and R. Marcus (1991). Clinical and anthropometric correlates of bone mineral acquisition in healthy adolescent girls. J. Clin. Endocrinol. Metab. 73: 1332-1339.

Kleerekoper, M., K. Tolia, and A.M. Parfitt (1981). Nutritional, endocrine, and demographic aspects of osteoporosis. Orthop. Clin. North Am. 12: 547-558.

Krabbe, S., and C. Christiansen (1984). Longitudinal study of calcium metabolism in male puberty. I. Bone mineral content, and serum levels of alkaline phosphatase, phosphate and calcium. Acta. Paediatr. Scand. 73: 745-749.

Krabbe, S., C. Christiansen, P. Rodbro, and I. Transbol (1979). Effect of puberty on rates of bone growth and mineralization. Arch. Dis. Child. 54: 950-953.

Krabbe, S., L. Hummer, and C. Christiansen (1984). Longitudinal study of calcium metabolism in male puberty. II. Relationship between mineralization and serum testosterone. Acta Paediatr. Scand. 73: 750-755.

Kramahoft, M., and S. Bodtker (1988). Epidemology of distal forearm fractures in Danish children. Acta Orthop. Scand. 59: 557-559.

Kroger, H., A. Kotaniemi, L. Kroger, and E. Alhava. (1993). Development of bone mass and bone density of the spine and femoral neck – a prospective study of 65 children and adolescents. Bone Miner. 23:171-182.

Kroger, H., A. Kotaniemi, P. Vainio, and E. Alhava (1992). Bone densitometry of the spine and femur in children by dual-energy x-ray absorptiometry. Bone Miner. 17: 75-85.

Laitinen, K., M. Valimaki, and P. Keto (1991). Bone mineral density measured by dual-energy x-ray absorptiometry in healthy Finnish women. Calcif. Tissue Int. 48: 224-231.

Landin, L., and B. Nilsson (1983). Bone mineral content in children with fractures. Clin. Orthop. 178: 292-296.

Landin, L.A. (1983). Fracture patterns in children. Acta Orthop. Scand. 54 (Suppl. 202): 1-63.

Li, J-Y., B.L. Specker, M.L. Ho, and R.C. Tsang (1989). Bone mineral content in Black and White children 1 to 6 years of age. A.J.D.C. 143: 1346-1349.

Lu, P.W., J.N. Briody, G.D. Ogle, K.Morley, I.R.J. Humphries, J. Allen, R. Howman-Giles, D. Sillence, and C.T. Cowell (1994). Bone mineral density of total body, spine, and femoral neck in children and young adults: a cross-sectional and longitudinal study. J. Bone Miner. Res. 9: 1451-1458.

Marcus, R., C. Cann, P. Mudvig, J. Minkoff, M. Goddard, M. Bayer, M. Martin, L. Gaudiani, W. Haskell, and H. Genant (1985). Menstrual function and bone mass in elite woman distance runners. Ann. Intern. Med. 102:158-163.

Matkovic, V., D. Fontana, C. Tominac, P. Goel, and C.H. Chestnut III (1990). Factors that influence peak bone mass formation: a study of calcium balance and the inheritance of bone mass in adolescent females. Am. J. Clin. Nutr. 52: 878-888.

Mazess, R.B., and H.S. Barden (1991). Bone density in premenopausal women: effects of age, dietary intake, physical activity, smoking and birth-control pills. Am. J. Clin. Nutr. 53:132-142.

Mazess, R.B., and H.M. Wahner (1988). Nuclear medicine and densitometry. In: B. L. Riggs and L.J. Melton, III (eds.) Osteoporosis: Etiology, Diagnosis, and Management. New York: Raven Press, pp. 251-295.

McCormick, D.P., S.W.Ponder, H.D.Fawcett, and J.L. Palmer (1991). Spinal bone mineral density in 335 normal and obese children and adolescents: evidence for ethnic and sex differences. J. Bone Miner. Res. 6: 507-513.

Melton, L.J. (1988). Epidemiology of fractures. In: B.L. Riggs & L.J. Melton, III (eds) Osteoporosis: Etiology, Diagnosis, and Management. New York: Raven Press, pp. 133-154.

Miller, J.Z., C.W. Slemenda, F.J. Meaney, T. K. Reister, S. Hui, and C.C. Johnston (1991). The relationship of bone mineral density and anthropometric variables in healthy male and female children. Bone Miner. 14: 137-152.

Pacifici, R., R. Rupich, I. Vered, K.C. Fisher, M. Griffin, N. Susman, and L.V. Avioli (1988). Dual energy radiography (DER): a preliminary comparative study. Calcif. Tissue Int. 43: 189-191.

Parfitt, A.M. (1988). Bone remodelling: Relationship to the amount and structure of bone, and the pathogenesis and prevention of fractures. In: R.L. Riggs and L.J. Melton, III (eds.) Osteoporosis: Etiology, Diagnosis, and Management. New York: Raven Press, pp. 45-93.

Parfitt, A.M. (1994). The two faces of growth: Benefits and risks to bone integrity. Osteop. Int. 4: 382-398.

Ponder, S.W., D.P. McCormick, D.Fawcett, J.L. Palmer, M.G. McKernan, and B.H. Brouhard (1990). Spinal bone mineral density in children aged 5.00 through 11.99 years. A.J.D.C. 144: 1346-1348.

Rice, S., C.J.R. Blimkie, C.E. Webber, D. Levy, J. Martin, D. Parker, and C.L. Gordon (1993). Correlates and determinants of bone mineral content and density in healthy adolescent girls. Can. J. Physiol. Pharmacol. 71: 923-930.

Rico, H., M. Vevilla, E.R. Hernandez, L.F. Villa, and M. Alverez del Buergo (1992). Sex differences in the acquisition of total bone mineral mass peak assessed through dual-energy x-ray absorptiometry. Calcif. Tissue Int. 51: 251-254.

Riis, B.J., S. Krabbe, C. Christiansen, B.D. Catherwood, and L.J. Deftos (1985). Bone turn-over in male puberty: a longitudinal study. Calcif. Tissue Int. 37: 213-217.

Robinson, T.L., C. Snow-Harter, D.R. Taaffe, D. Gillis, J. Shaw, and R. Marcus (1995). Gymnasts exhibit higher bone mass than runners despite similar prevalence of amenor-rhea and oligomenorrhea. J. Bone Miner. Res. 10: 26-35.

Rodin, A., B. Murby, M.A. Smith, M. Caleffi, I Fentiman, M.G. Chapman, and I. Fogelman (1990). Premenopausal bone loss in the lumbar spine and neck of femur: a study of 225 caucasian women. Bone 11: 1-5.

Rubin, K., V. Schirduan, P. Gendreau, M. Sarfarazi, R. Mendola, and G. Dalsky (1993). Pre-dictors of axial and peripheral bone mineral density in healthy children and adolescents, with special attention to the role of puberty. J. Pediatr. 123:863-870.

Sentipal, J., G.M. Wardlaw, J. Mahan, and V. Matkovic (1991). Influence of calcium intake and growth indexes on vertebral bone mineral density in young females. Am. J. Clin. Nutr. 54: 425-428.

Shipp, C.C., P.S. Berger, M.S. Dechr, and B. Dawson-Hughes (1988). Precision of dual-pho-ton absorptiometry. Calcif. Tissue Int. 42: 287-292.

Slemenda, C.W., T.K. Reister, J.Z. Miller, J.C. Christian, and C.C. Johnston Jr.(1994). Influ-ences on skeletal mineralization in children and adolescents: Evidence for varying effects of sexual maturation and physical activity. J. Pediatr. 125:201-207.

Smith, R. (1980). Idiopathic osteoporosis in the young. J. Bone Joint Surg. (Br.) 62: 417-427.

Southard, R.N., J.D. Morris, J.D. Mahan, J.R. Hayes, M.A. Torch, A. Sommer, and W.B. Zipf (1991). Bone mass in healthy children: measurement with quantitative DXA. Radiology 179:735-738.

Sugimoto, T., M. Nishino, T. Tsunenari, M. Kawakatsu, K. Shimogaki, Y. Fujii, H. Negishi, M. Tsutsumi, M. Fukase, and K. Chihara (1994). Radial bone mineral content of normal Japanese infants and prepubertal children: influence of age, sex, and body size. Bone Mi-ner. 24: 189-200.

Teitelbaum, S.L. (1993). Skeletal growth and development. In: M.J. Favus (ed.) Primer on the Metabolic Bone Diseases and Disorders of Mineral Metabolism. Second Edition. New York: Raven Press, pp. 7-11.

Theintz, G., B. Buchs, R. Rizzoli, D. Slosman, H. Clavien, P.C. Sizonenko, and J.-PH Bon-jour (1992). Longitudinal monitoring of bone mass accumulation in healthy adolescents: Evidence for a marked reduction after 16 years of age at the levels of lumbar spine and fe-moral neck in female subjects. J. Clin. Endocrinol. Metab. 75: 1060-1065.

Thomas K.A., S.D. Cook, J.T. Bennett, T.S. Whitecloud III, and J.C. Rice (1991). Femoral neck and lumbar spine bone mineral densities in a normal population 3-20 years of age. J. Pediatr. Orthop. 11:48-58.

Tothill, P. (1989). Methods of bone mineral measurement. Phys. Med. Biol. 34: 543-572.

Warren, M.P., J. Brooks-Gunn, R.P. Fox, C.Lancelot, D. Newman, and W.G. Hamilton (1991). Lack of bone accretion and amenorrhea: evidence for a relative osteopenia in weight-bearing bones. J. Clin. Endocrinol. Metab. 72: 847-853.

White, C.M., A.C. Hergenroeder, and W.J. Klish (1992). Bone mineral density in 15- to 21-year-old eumenorrheic and amenorrheic subjects. A.J.D.C. 146: 31-35.

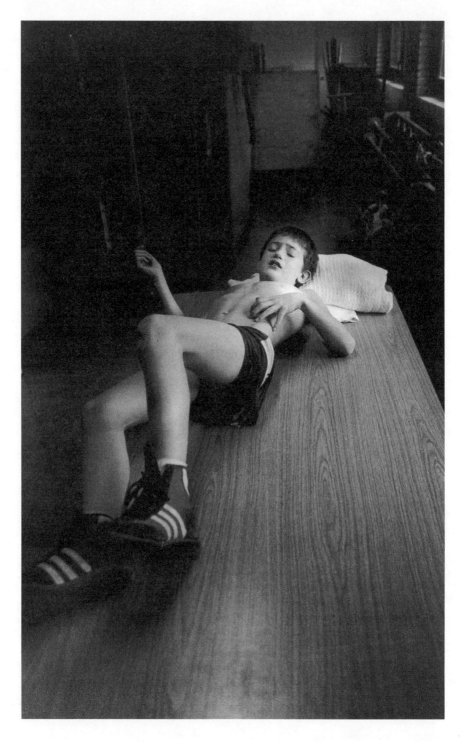

Chapter 10

Skeletal Development in Children and Adolescents and the Relations with Physical Activity

Han C. G. Kemper

Introduction

In this article a review will be given about the developmental aspects of the skeleton during growth of children and the relations between physical activity and bone mass during youth.

After a short historical description of the methods used in the past, from simple whole body measurements, more specific anthropometrical methods, radiographic measurements and more quantitative measurements of skeletal mass will be reviewed.

The second part is concerned with a literature survey about the natural course of skeletal development, emphasizing differences in early and late maturing children, the changes in bone mineral density during growth, and the age period that the maximal bone mineral density will be reached. This will be illustrated with results from the Amsterdam Growth and Health study (Kemper, 1985).

The last section is devoted to the specific effects of life-style of youth on the skeletal development: A meta-analysis about the effects of calcium intake in the diet (Welten et al., 1995) reveals the influence on bone mass and recent results from the Amsterdam Growth and Health Study (Kemper, 1995) compare the differential effects of energetic and biomechanic components of habitual physical activities during youth on the bone mineral density of males and females at age 28.

Methods of skeletal development assesment

Physical growth and development have been extensively investigated from prenatal growth to birth, and from postnatal growth to adulthood by many longitudinal studies all over the world. Tanner's monograph "A history of the study of human growth" is a main source (1981), together with the "Origins of the study of human growth" by Boyd (1980) and the unfinished work left by Richard E. Scammon, the late professor in anatomy at the University of Minnesota.

Anthropometrics

The methods first used are mainly based on anthropometric measurements of total body dimensions such as body height and body weight or body segments (sitting height, arm- and leg length and width measurements (shoulder and hip) (Weiner and Lourie, 1969).

Von Döbeln (1959 and 1964) proposed a measure for estimation of the skeletal weight from height and four breadth measurements (left and right femur condyli and radio-ulnar width). This sounds good as long as it is used for estimating total weight of bone mass in comparison with estimates of muscle and fat mass estimated by skinfolds and circumferences in combination with height and weight. In the Netherlands, however, this concept is used to correct the body weight to body height relationship: The Dutch Heart Foundation constructed a scale ("waag-schaal") based on the Quetelet Index or Body Mass Index (QI or BMI: weight/height^2) that included the possibility of correcting the ideal body weight on the basis of the breadth of the femur condyle. This is a misuse of the skeletal component because it makes adjustments for the least variant of the three component model of body composition with lean and fat mass being the other components. In a health promotion policy it gives the overweight people an excuse to correct their own body weight towards a more favorable weight profile or status.

The use of BMI is widely used because it is easy to use (only height and weight are needed) and it is also accepted as a measure of obesity in both children and adults. It more or less assumes, however, that the weight of fat mass is the most variant component and that the weight of muscle mass (as the skeletal weight) remains invariant in the determination of total body weight. This may be valid in a normal population and BMI can be seen as a rough estimate of average fatness in large samples. However, the more direct measurement from skinfolds or with other techniques such as densitometry (underwater weighing) avoid bias in people with different body proportions (small children and muscular people) (Lohman, 1992).

Radiographics

On November 1895, over a hundred years ago, the German physicist Wilhelm Conrad Röntgen discovered gamma radiation and demonstrated a radiogram showing the bones of his own hand. He called this X radiation. The famous anatomist Albert von Kölliker connected Röntgen's name to this kind of radiation.

Since then, X rays are widely used in medicine for detection of infectious diseases, pathologic neoplasmata and traumatology.

A whole other field of applying radiographics is the use of skeletal growth and development as a measure of biological age. Skeletal maturation begins as a process when rudiments of bones appear during embryonic life and is completed when skeletal form becomes comparatively stable in young adulthood. During maturation there are increases in the types and numbers of specialized cells, including cartilage and fibrous tissue cells that form part of a bone (Roche et al., 1988). In 1950 Greulich and Pyle published their radiographic atlas of skeletal development of the hand and wrist with a second edition in 1959. Roche et al. (1975) from his Fels Longitudinal Study used the knee joint as bones of interest for determination of skeletal maturation (Roche-Wainer-Thissen method, RWT). Most assessments of skeletal maturity are made from radiographs of the hand-wrist, because this site has considerable advantages over other parts of the skeleton. These advantages stem from the little irradiation required, the ease of radiographic positioning, and the large number of bones included in the area. Therefore, the RWT method using the knee joint as a biological indicator (Roche, Wainer and Thissen, 1975) was extended with the hand-wrist (Fels) method. In Europe, Tanner et al. from the Institute of Child Health in London published their TW2 method in 1975, also using X-ray photographs of the left hand including 20 bones of the hand and wrist.

All these skeletal maturity scales are used to estimate the developmental or biological age of children, correcting for children who mature faster or slower than the average child with the same calendar age. In pediatrics it can be used to predict adult height of children (mostly girls) who or whose parents expect that they will end up very tall, and consider to intervene in their growth by using hormones to close their endplates earlier.

In the field of growth and development, a distinction can be made between two fundamentally different types of ages: chronological age (CA) and biological age (BA). CA refers to the number of years a person lived since birth. As an indicator of biological maturity it has a number of shortcomings, and this is especially true during the pubertal years, due to the wide variation in the onset of pubertal changes (10-16 years CA). The BA of a child provides us with an improved measure of maturation: it measures the progress along the road of life anatomically, physiologically and mentally (Cheek, 1968). This can be illustrated by a group of Danish girls that were photographed in the gymnasium and were arranged in two ways: first according to their CA, and second according their BA. As can be seen from figure 1 (page 142), the height of these girls corresponds quite nicely with their BA, but not with their CA.

Single events to measure BA that have been used frequently are: age of menarche in girls (Jones 1949, Marshall, 1978, Prader 1978), body structure development index (Koinzer et al., 1981, Meszaros et al., 1985), and age of peak height velocity (Carron, Bailey 1974, Kobayashi et al., 1978, Mirwald et al., 1981, Rutenfranz et al., 1982, Cunningham et al., 1984). Series of consecutive events such as calcification stages of long and short bones, as described before, or of teeth (Lewis and Garn 1960) have been proposed as more refined estimators of maturity (Prahl-Andersen and Roede 1979). In the Amsterdam growth and health study, both single measurements (menarche and peak height velocity) and serial measurements of the skeletal maturity of the hand and wrist (TW2 method) were used (Kemper and Verschuur, 1981). We measured BA of a group of boys and girls annually during four years starting with a CA of 13. On the basis of a comparison of this longitudinal measurement of BA with CA, fast and late maturers were discerned (Kemper et al., 1987). The results showed that even during these serial measurements of skeletal age there are boys and girls who are slow maturers at CA of 13 but fast maturers at age 16 (Fig 2 page 143).

Figure 1: A group of Danish girls arranged according to calendar age (bottom) and biological age (top). Personal communication with O. Lammert.

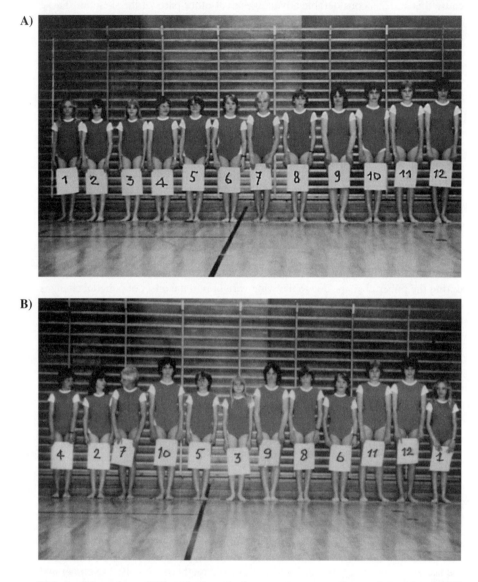

This questions the validity of using single measurements of maturity such as PHV as an alternative of CA, when regrouping and re-analyzing longitudinal data of anthropometry and physiological functions relative to years before or after the age of menarche and peak height velocity (Beunen, Malina 1991).

The advantage of rapid maturers (RM) with respect to slow maturers (SM) in many sports is that during puberty their greater body height and weight is of importance for their performance, especially in contact sport games such as soccer

Figure 2: The relation between calendar age and biological age in four girls (left) and four boys (right) measured in 4 consecutive years.

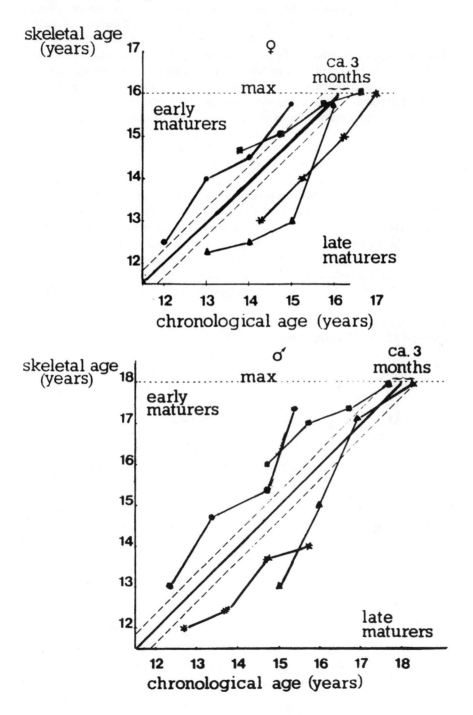

and handball, and individual sports like high jump or shot put. But this is certainly not the case at the end of maturation. We found that body height at full maturity was not different between rapid and slow maturers. This was also the case in physiological parameters such as maximal oxygen uptake and maximal isometric strength (Kemper et al., 1986). Further analysis showed that there was a distinct difference in the percentage of fat mass between rapid and slow maturers; the slow maturers were significantly leaner than the rapid maturers, and this was the case from the start of pubertal growth (CA 12-13 years) until the end of puberty (CA 16-18). But recently, Van Lenthe showed in the same subjects, that also at CA of 27 years, the rapid maturers were fatter than the slow maturers in both sexes (figure 3 and 4).

The consequences of the higher fat mass in the rapid maturers was that they showed significantly lower maximal oxygen uptake (VO_2max/BM) and maximal isometric strength (Fmax/BM) in relation to their body mass.

In the Amsterdam Growth and Health Study, we also monitored life styles like habitual food intake (Post et al., 1993) and physical activity (Kemper et al., 1994). From these data we could search into the possible causes of these differences between rapid and slow maturers. It appeared that between the ages of 13 and 22 years, the RMs in both sexes consumed less energy and less protein, but also spent less time and energy in physical activity than the SMs. A slow maturation seems,

Figure 3: Development of sum of 4 skinfolds in rapid and slow maturing girls between 13 and 27 years of age.

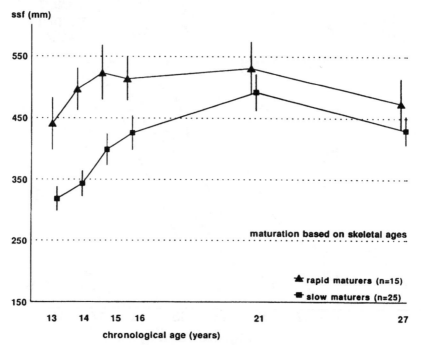

Figure 4: Development of sum of 4 skinfolds in rapid and slow maturing boys between 13 and 27 years of age.

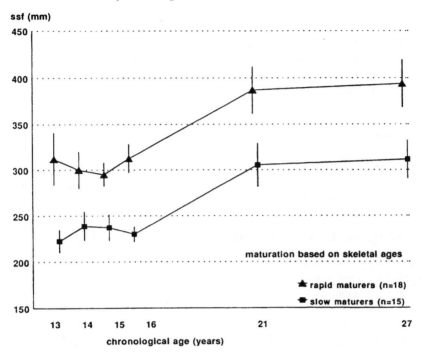

therefore, to coincide with a more appropriate energy balance during adolescence. This was exactly one of the speculations of Garn et al. (1968) who found in about 16,000 white women, that RMs are fatter than SMs. The mechanisms for these differences are not known, but it can be hypothesized that a rapid maturation causes a socializing away from a physical active life style, resulting in an early dropping out from sport activities during adolescence.

Dual Energy X-ray Absorptiometry (DEXA)
While radiographs cannot easily quantify bone density (because 30% of it has to be lost before it is seen on X-ray), recent technical advances have made it possible to measure bone mass by energy absorption from gamma radiation in the bone. DEXA is now the most precise and widely used method of assessing bone density, and the preferred method because scanning time is shorter than with dual photon absorptiometry (DPA), resolution is improved, and measurements can be made in the spine, femoral neck, forearm and for the total body.

From the DEXA method, two measures are calculated: the bone mineral content (BMC) and the bone mineral density (BMD). The BMC is the mass of minerals in the selected bone in grams, and the BMD is the mass divided by the area of the selected bone (gram x cm^{-2}). This is therefore called area density.

Whereas in growth studies bones not only increase their area but also their volume, these size changes influence the areal BMD. Therefore, attempts have been made to correct for this bone size effect by an additional measure of bone mineral apparent density (BMAD).

Quantitative Computed Tomography (QCT)

QCT systems have been adapted for estimation of bone mineral content allowing cortical bone to be separated from trabecular bone. Furthermore, it provides us with a true measure of total, cortical or trabecular bone mineral volumetric density (mg x mm^{-3}). However, the equipment is more expensive, and exposes patients to high radiation doses. A peripheral QCT system is now available for the forearm with a lower dose of radiation.

Ultrasound

Ultrasound measurements have been available since 1984 for the calcaneus, and have the potential for wide-spread clinical applications.

Development of bone mass during growth

Not much is known about the exact timing of the calendar or biological age at which the maximal amount of bone mass is reached. Therefore, the literature is reviewed firstly about the bone development in boys and girls before puberty. Secondly, an estimation is made about the importance of the pubertal period in the total development of bone mass. Thirdly, the question about the age at which maximal or peak bone mineral density occurs in males and females is addressed.

Development of bone density before puberty

The six cross-sectional studies (Gilsanz et al., 1988, Glastre et al., 1990, Gordon et al., 1991, Southard et al., 1991, Bonjour et al., 1991 and Geusens et al., 1991) and the only longitudinal study of Theintz et al. (1992) conclude that there is not much sex difference in bone density before puberty. All studies measured at the lumbar spine, two also at the femur, and only Geusens et al. (1991) measured the total body BMD. Although a clear trend is found in all of the above mentioned studies of a gradual increase in BMD, it is not possible to make a more quantitative estimation of the proportional contribution to the total adult BMD.

Development of bone density during puberty

The relative short period of life of the pubertal stage of boys and girls of about 3 to 5 years seems to be a very important one for the development of bone mass. In table 1, the percentage increase in BMD in girls varies between 17 and 70%, and in boys, between 11 and 75% of total adult values. The data are gathered from 7 cross-sectional studies (Gilsanz et al., 1988, Glastre et al., 1990, Geusens et al., 1991, Gordon et al., 1991, Bonjour et al., 1991, Grimston et al., 1992 and Riis et al., 1985).

Apart from factors like differences in classification of pubertal stages, rapid and slow maturation and regional differences, the wide variation can be attributed to

Table 1: Overview of seven studies that estimated the percentage of BMD accrued in boys and girls during their pubertal years.

Lumbar Spine	Method	% increase in girls	% increase in boys
Gilsanz et al, 1988	QCT	17%	-
Glastre et al, 1990	DXA	41%	-
Geusens et al, 1991	DXA	70%	75%
Gordon et al, 1991	DXA	38%	11%
Bonjour et al, 1991	DXA	51%	53%
Grimston et al, 1992	DXA	48%	48%
Radial:			
Riis et al, 1991	DXA	-	31%

the DEXA method. Determination of BMD by projectional methods like DEXA provide areal densities (g x cm^{-2}) which are confounded by size changes accompanying growth. A cube of bone that is twice as big as a cube of bone with the same BMD, results in twice as high areal BMD when it is scanned by DEXA (Bailey et al., 1993). This dimensional consideration explains why Gilsanz et al. (1988) shows the lowest increase of 15%, since this was the only study that used QCT to measure BMD and this method provides a real volumetric BMD.

The BMD changes during the growth period that are reported, indicating that 50% of BMD is accrued around puberty, must be doubted seriously. During this period, however, there is a very large gain in bone mass, as reflected in BMC.

Age at which peak bone mineral density (PBMD) is reached
Most of the anatomical structures and physiological functions such as muscle mass, cardio-respiratory functions, immune system and central nervous system show a typical pattern over time. This is characterized by a steep increase during the growth period until the age of 20 years, and thereafter a much slower decrease and gradual decline during aging (Kemper and Binkhorst 1993). This pattern implies that there is a point of time or period that the human functions reach their maximal capacities. At the occasion of the Wolff memorial lecture at the ACSM conference in Indianapolis in 1994, Barbara Drinkwater (personal communication) showed the hypothetical curves of boys and girls of BMD, suggesting that BMD increases from 0.7 g x cm^{-2} at age 4 up to 1.3-1.4 g x cm^{-2} at age 20 (figure 5 page 148).

A closer look into the literature provided us with seven valid cross-sectional studies (Gilsanz et al., 1988, Buchanan et al., 1988, Glastre et al., 1990, Geusens et

Figure 5: Developmental curves of BMD in both boys and girls from birth to adulthood by Drinkwater (pers. communication).

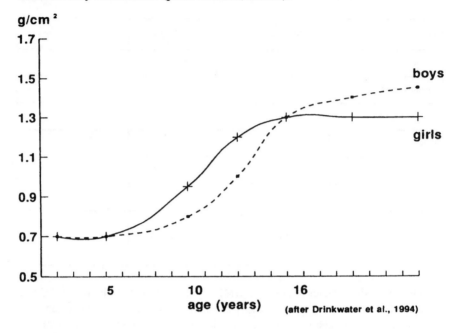

al., 1991, Bonjour et al., 1991, Rico et al., 1992, Teegarden et al., 1995). They report an age period of reaching PBMD in females (7 studies) between 16 and 26 and in boys (3 studies) between 16 and 25 years.

Two valid longitudinal studies investigated the development of BMD and PBMD and both of them used female subjects. Both studies, Davies et al. (1990) with a follow-up of 4 years and Recker et al. (1992) with a follow-up of 5 years, show very clearly that at least in females the age of PBMD is not before 20 years of age: both lumbar, radial and total BMD reach their highest values in the late twenties. This is recently confirmed by Teegarden et al. (1995) showing that in women 99% of total body BMD is attained by age 22 and 99% of total BMC at age 26 (figure 6).

It can be concluded that PBMD in females will be reached relatively late compared to other physiological functions: not in the late teens but in the early or late twenties.

Another question is if there is a difference in PBMD in males and females who are rapid or slow maturers during their teens. Rapid maturation coincides with a relative longer exposure to sex specific hormones than slow maturation. Estrogen levels in girls and testosterone levels in boys seem to be related to bone mass development. In the Amsterdam Growth and Health Study we selected RMs and SMs on the basis of four annual measurements of skeletal age of the hand and wrist between the age of 12 and 17 years, and compared the BMD at age 27-29

Figure 6: Total body bone mineral content (TBBMC) and total body bone mineral density (TBBMD) plotted against calendar age in women (after Teegarden et al., 1995).

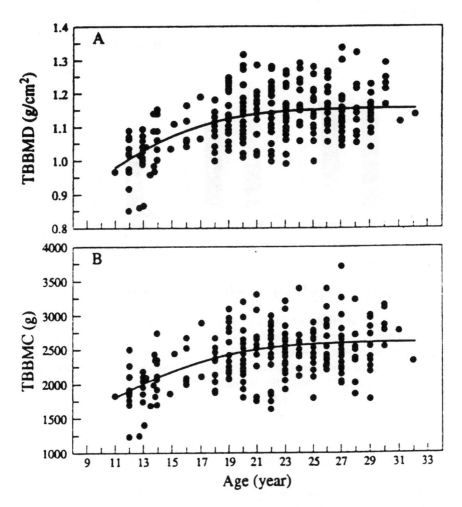

years of the lumbar spine, femoral neck and distal radius (figure 7 page 150). The results show clearly that at adult age in both sexes the BMD at none of the three selected sides is significantly different between RMs and LMs. This is in contrast with earlier findings of Dhuper et al. (1990), Riis et al. (1985) and Finkelstein et al. (1992) who found lower BMD in SMs compared to RMs. These studies, however, were no longitudinal studies, did not measure BMD at adult age, and did not establish rapid or slow maturation by skeletal age over a period of 4 years.

Figure 7: Bone mineral density in rapid (n=33) and slow maturers (n=40) measured at age between 27 and 29 years. No significance (p<0.05) could be demonstrated at the lumbar spine, femoral neck or distal radius in both sexes.

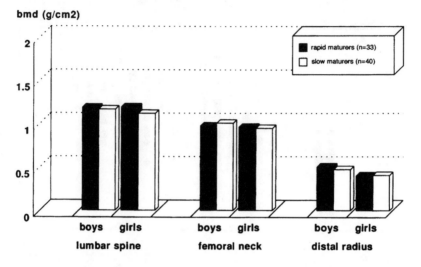

Effects of lifestyle on skeletal development

It is widely accepted that a healthy life-style has beneficial effects on the development and maintenance of the skeleton. Nutrition and physical activity are thought to be the more important aspects of life-style. Nutrition may be an important determinant of bone mass with calcium as the most important nutrient (Matkovic et al., 1990, Sentipal et al., 1991). For physical activity, it is still uncertain which are the most important influences, e.g. type, intensity, duration or frequency of activity (Snow-Harter and Marcus, 1991, Kemper et al., 1995).

Effects of calcium intake

Recently Welten et al. (1995) published a meta-analysis of the effect of calcium intake on bone mass in young and middle aged females, and males to find a direct relationship between dietary calcium and bone mass. From a total of 33 eligible studies identified in the literature, 27 were cross-sectional, 2 longitudinal and 4 intervention studies. The summary effect measures were calculated separately for the cross-sectional, the longitudinal and the intervention studies by first weighing the mean effects by sample size and then averaging. For each weighted summary measure of effect, a 95% confidence interval (95% CI) was given (table 2).

The results of the 18 cross-sectional studies with more than 2500 females showed a significant r of 0.13 as well as a significant partial of 0.08. In males (n~200), the results were not significant. The 4 intervention studies found that calcium supplementation of about 1000 mg per day in woman (n~200) can prevent the loss of 1% of bone at all bone sites except in the ulna.

Table 2: Weighted summary effect measures of calcium intake on bone mineral mass: In the cross-sectional and longitudinal studies the effect measures are the Pearson product moment correlations (r) and the partial correlations (partial), and in the intervention studies the percentage difference (PERDIF) in yearly bone loss between the calcium supplemented and the control group.

Effect measure	n	Mean	Weighted mean	95%-CI
		Cross-sectional studies, females		
r	2550 (18)	0.12	0.13	(0.09; 0.16)
partial r	2493 (18)	0.08	0.08	(0.05; 0.12)
		Cross-sectional studies, males		
r	273 (2)	0.02	0.01	(-0.11; 0.13)
partial r	195 (2)	0.02	0.02	(-0.12; 0.16)
		Longitudinal studies, females		
r	396 (2)	0.06	0.04	(-0.06; 0.14)
partial r	0 (0)	—	—	—
		Intervention studies, females		
PERDIF	193 (4)	1.11	1.32	(1.21; 1.42)

From this analysis it can be concluded that calcium intake is positively associated with bone mass in premenopausal females. This association is fairly consistent across different study designs and is strengthened by the fact that the results are only based on studies with a high methodological quality. The available data are not adequate to state the same conclusion for males: There are very few studies (2 cross-sectional, 2 longitudinal and no intervention) and the weighted summary effects of calcium intake upon BMD are not statistically significant (p> 0.05).

Probably one of the factors that influences the effect of dietary calcium is the level of calcium intake in the different populations. In the Netherlands, boys and girls from the age of 13 years have relatively high calcium intakes that meet or are well above recommended daily intake (Kemper et al., 1995), and therefore, no significant effects could be demonstrated. This is in contrast with French children and adolescents (Ruiz et al., 1995), who have low calcium intakes and therefore, the spontaneous calcium intake is significantly related to BMD, especially at the lumbar site (fig 8 page 152).

Figure 8: Relationship between vertebral BMD and dietary calcium intake in 81 girls and 70 boys (after Ruiz et al., 1995)

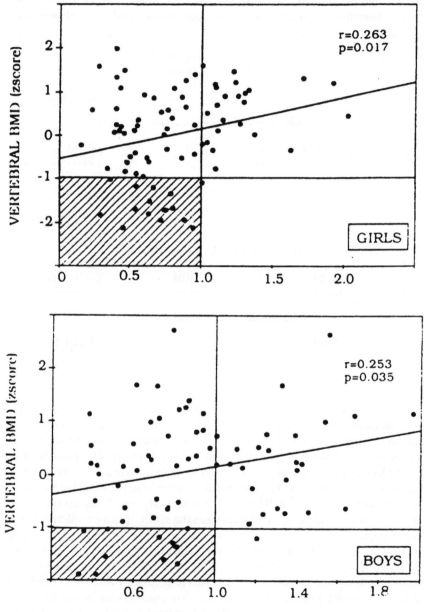

Effects of physical activity

Although the positive effect of physical activity on bone mass often has been con-firmed, there are still some uncertainties about the mechanism which leads to an increase in BMD. Animal experiments in which mechanical loads of various cycles were applied to bones showed that the osteogenic response to dynamic loading is soon i.e. after 36 repetitions, saturated (Rubin et al., 1984, Lanyon, 1992). In human epidemiological studies, physical activities are estimated on the basis of intensity (as a percentage of maximal oxygen uptake or maximal heart rate) and duration (minutes per day or week), emphasizing the energetic com-ponents of the physical activities. If the effect of load magnitude should outweigh cycle number, a reasonable hypothesis should be that physical activities with peak strain (high loads with few repetitions) have a greater effect on bone mass than en-durance activities (high number of repetitions and low loads).

In the Amsterdam Growth and Health Longitudinal Study (Kemper 1995) we monitored daily physical activity from age 12 until age 29 in a group of 182 males and females. At the mean age of 28 years a single measurement of BMD was measured at three sites: the lumbar region, femoral neck and proximal radius by DEXA.

The physical activity pattern was measured six times in the foregoing years by a cross-check interview (Verschuur 1987). All activities in the three months prece-ding the interview were considered: transportation, organized sports, jobs, school physical education, leisure time activities, gardening, stair climbing etc.

To answer the question what the most important factor is for bone mass develop-ment during youth, we scored the physical activity data in two different ways: (1) emphasizing the energetic components by weighting the metabolic intensity (METs) and duration (minutes per week)and (2) emphasizing the biomechanical components by weighting the peak strain (i.e. the ground reaction forces as a multiple of body weight) irrespective of the frequency and the duration of the activity.

In table 3 (page 154), examples of the weighted MET-scores and in table 4 of the weighted peak strain scores are given.

The contrasts between both scoring methods can be shown in two examples of sport activities: swimming is scored as high energy (3) and low peak strain (0), while volleyball is scored as low energy (1) and high peak strain (3).

The habitual physical activity scores were calculated for each subject over three time periods: the adolescent period (four annual measurements between 13 and 17 years of age), the young adult period (two measurements between 17 and 22 years of age), and the adult period (two measurements between 22 and 28 years of age).

Linear regression analysis were performed to analyze the relation between BMD at age 28 and the physical activity scores over three foregoing periods. The physical activity scores were entered in the regression model as independent vari-ables, and gender was added to the model as a covariate.

In figure 9, 10 (page 155) and 11 (page 156), the standard regression coefficients of lumbar BMD, hip BMD and radius BMD, respectively, are given for the MET-score and the peak scores, and for the three different periods.

Table 3: Scoring of the energetic component of habitual physical activities by weighting MET-scores

ACTIVITIES	INTENSITY LEVEL	EXAMPLES	SCORE
heavy	> 10 MET's	Track and field (track), swimming, basketball, rowing	3
medium heavy	7 - 10 MET's	stair climbing, skating, gymnastics, track and field (field), tennis	2
light	4 - 7 MET's	weightlifting, volleyball, bicycling, horseback riding, sailing	1
very light	< 4 MET's	walking, yoga, bowling	0

SUMSCORE = Σ x time

Table 4: Scoring of the biomechanical component of habitual physical activities by weighting the peak strain scores

ACTIVITIES	GROUND REACTION FORCES (x body-weight)	EXAMPLES	SCORE
jumping	5 - 10	volleyball, basketball, gymnastics	3
turning, sprinting, explosive	3 - 5	track and field (field) soccer, tennis, judo, ballet, stairclimbing	2
running, loaded walking	1 - 3	track and field (track), house cleaning, horseback riding, skating, rowing	1
strolling, sitting, standing	0.5 - 1	swimming, car driving, bicycling, sailing, remedial gym	0

SUMSCORE = Σ

The results show that as the time period over which the physical activity scores were taken, came closer to the BMD measurement at age 28, the more important became the peak component of physical activity. For this biomechanical component of physical activity, the explained variance of BMD increased from 2% during adolescence to 13 % in adulthood. For the energetic component of physical activity the explained variance on the other hand decreased from 6% during adolescence to 1% in adulthood. These relations were found for both sexes and for both lumbar and femoral neck BMD. For the distal radius BMD, there were as expected, no significant relations with either physical activity scores.

Figure 9: The relationship of BMD in the lumbar spine at age 28 years with energetic physical activity (MET-score) and peak strain physical activity (Peak-score) during three different preceding periods in 182 males and females from the Amsterdam Growth and Health Study

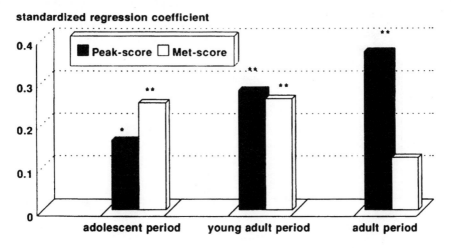

Figure 10: The relationship of BMD in the femoral neck at age 28 years with energetic physical activity (Met-score) and peak strain physical activity (Peak-score) during three different preceding periods in 182 males and females from the Amsterdam Growth and Health Study

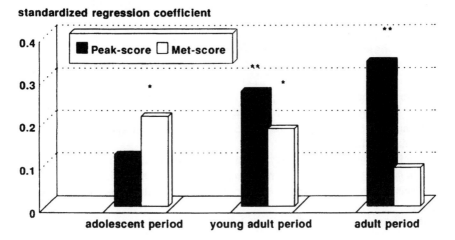

From these results it can be concluded that habitual physical activity measured as peak strain has in both sexes a better osteogenic effect than physical activity measured as metabolic rate. This confirms the hypothesis that the biomechanical strain component not only in animal experiments but also in young healthy people is a

Figure 11: The relationship of BMD in the distal radius at age 28 years with energetic physical activity (MET-score) and peak strain physical activity (Peak-score) during three different preceding periods in 182 males and females from the Amsterdam Growth and Health Study

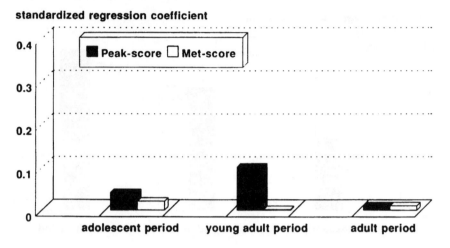

more important factor for developing and maintaining a high peak bone mineral density in the weight bearing parts of the human skeleton. This differential effect of biomechanic and energetic aspects of physical activity has to be considered in the promotion of exercise programs for the prevention of different chronic diseases.

Conclusions

Conclusions about the natural course of skeletal development
Before the age of puberty no clear differences in BMD between boys and girls are demonstrated.

During the pubertal growth spurt it is likely that the increase in BMD on the average is about 20% of total BMD increase.

Women reach their peak BMD between the early and late twenties, while there are no data available for males.

Rapid and slow maturation seem to have a significant effect on fat mass and lifestyle at (young) adult age: rapid maturing boys and girls have higher fat mass and their energy intake compared to energy expenditure results into a positive energy balance.

Maturation rate has no effect on peak BMD.

Conclusions about the effects of life-style on skeletal development
Recent (quasi) experimental research indicates that physical activity can have beneficial effects on site specific BMD.

The dietary calcium intake enhances BMD in girls and premenopausal females if the intake levels are below recommendations.

Physical activity measured as peak strain has a better osteogenic effect in both sexes than physical activity measured as energy expenditure.

The energetic effects on peak BMD (measured at age 28) is most pronounced during adolescence, and the peak strain effects are more important in the current adult period.

Acknowledgment:
The author expresses his gratitude to the subjects, who served in the Amsterdam Growth Study, the staff (W. van Mechelen, G.B. Post, J. Snel, J.W.R. Twisk, D.C. Welten, F.J. van Lenthe), who measured and calculated the longitudinal data and last but not least the institutions that granted us over the 15 years period (Prevention Fund, Dutch Heart Foundation, Ministry of Health, Wellbeing and Sport, Dairy Foundation on Nutrition and Health).

References

Bailey D, Drinkwater D, Faulkner R, McKay H. Proximal femur bone mineral changes in growing children: dimensional considerations. Ped Exerc Sci 5: 388, 1993

Beunen G, Malina R. Growth and physical performances related to the timing of the adolescent spurt. Exerc Sport Sci Rev 16: 503-541, 1988

Bonjour JF, Theintz G, Buchs B, Slosman D, Rizzoli R. Critical years and stages of puberty for spinal and femoral bone mass accumulation during adolescence. J Clin Endocrin Soc 73: 555-563, 1991

Boyd E. Origins of the study of human growth. University of Oregon Health Sciences Center Foundation, 1980

Buchanan JR, Meyers C, Lloyd T, Leuenberger P, Demers L. Determinants of peak trabecular bone density in women: the role of androgens, estrogen, and exercise. J Bone Min Res 3: 673-680, 1988a

Buchanan JR, Meyers C, Lloyd T, Greer RB III. Early vertebral trabecular bone loss in normal premenopausal women. J Bone Min res 3: 445-449, 1988b

Carron AV, Bailey DA. Strength development in boys from 10 through 16 years. Monogr Soc Res Child Dev 157: 39, 1974

Cunningham DA, Paterson DH, Blimkie CJR, Donner AP. Development of cardiorespiratory function in circumpubertal boys: a longitudinal study. J Appl Physiol 56: 302-307, 1984

Cheek B. Human growth: body composition, cell growth, energy and intelligence. Lea and Febiger, Philadelphia, 1968

Davies KM, Recker RR, Stegman MR, Heaney RP, Kimmel DB, Leist J. Calcium regulation and bone metabolism. Elsevier Science: 497-50, 1990

Dobeln W von. Anthropometric determination of fat-free body weight. Acta Med Scand 165: 37, 1959

Dobeln W von. Determination of body constituants. In: Occurrence, causes and prevention of overnutrition. G Blix (ed) Almquist and Wiksells, Uppsala, 1964

Dhuper S, Warren MP, Brooks-Gunn J, Fox R. Effect of hormonal status on bone density in adolescent girls. J Clin Endocrinol Metab 71: 1083-1088, 1990

Finkelstein JS, Neer RM, Biller BMK, Crawford JD, Klibanski A. Osteoporosis in men with a history of delayed puberty. NEJM 27: 600-603, 1992

Garn SM, La Velle M, Rosenberg KR, Hawthorne VM. Maturational timing as a factor in female fatness and obesity. Am J Clin Nutr 43: 879-883, 1986

Geusens P, Cantatore F, Nijs J, Proesmans W, Emma F, Dequeker J. Heterogenity of growth of bone in children at the spine, radius and total skeleton. Growth, Development and Aging 55: 249-256, 1991

Gilsanz V, Gibbons DT, Roe TF, Carlson M. Vertebral bone density in children: effect of puberty Radiology: 166: 847-850, 1988a

Gilsanz V, Gibbons DT, Carlson M. Peak trabecular vertebral density: a comparison of adolescent and adult females. Calcif Tissue Int 43: 260-262, 1988b

Glastre C, Braillon P, David L, Cochat P, Meunier PJ, Delmas PD. Measurement of bone mineral content of the lumbar spine by dual energy X-ray absorptiometry in normal children: correlations with growth parameters. J Clin Endocrinol and Metab 70: 1330-1333, 1990

Gordon CL, Halton JM, Atkinson SA, Webber CE. The contributions of growth and puberty to peak bone mass. Growth, Development and Aging 55: 257-262, 1991

Greulich W, Pyle SI. Radiographic atlas of skeletal development of the hand and wrist. Stanford Univ Press, Stanford, 1950 and 1959 (Sec edition)

Grimston SK, Morrison K, Harder JA, Hanley DA. Bone mineral density during puberty in Western Canadian children. Bone and Min Res 19: 85-96, 1992

Jones H, Priest JD, Hayes WC, Chinn Tichenor C, Nagel DA. Humeral hypertrophy in response to exercise 59-A: 204-208, 1977

Kemper HCG, Niemeyer C. The importance of a physically active life-style during youth of peak bone mass. In: New horizons in pediatric exercise, CJR Blimkie, O Bar-Or (eds) Human Kinetics, Champaign, Chapter 5: 77-95, 1995.

Kemper HCG, Welten DC, Twisk JWR. Reply on the letter to the editor of RP Heaney on weight-bearing activity during youth is a more important factor for peak bone mass than calcium intake. J Bone and Min Res 10, 1: 172-174, 1995

Kemper HCG, Binkhorst RA. Exercise and the physiological consequences of the aging process. In: JJF Schroots (ed) Aging, health and competence. Elsevier, Amsterdam, 6: 109-126, 1993

Kemper HCG, Post GB. Biological maturation is related to nutrient intake and physical activity during adolescence. Med Sci Sports Exercise 25: S92 abstract, 1993

Kemper HCG, Verschuur R, Ritmeester J-W. Maximal aerobic power in early and late maturing teenagers. In: Children and Exercise XII, J Rutenfranz, R Mocellin, F Klimt. Int Series on Sport Sciences vol 17, Human Kinetics, Champaign: 213-225, 1986

Kemper HCG, Verschuur R, Ritmeester J-W. Longitudinal development of growth and fitness in early and late maturing teenagers. Pediatrician 14: 219-225, 1987

Kemper HCG, Verschuur R. Maximal aerobic power in 13- and 14-year old teenagers in relation to biological age. Int J Sports Med 2: 97-100, 161-262, 1981

Kemper HCG (ed). Growth, Health and Fitness of Teenagers, longitudinal research in international perspective. Medicine and Sport Science (M Hebbelinck, ed), vol 20. Karger, Basel, 1985

Kemper HCG (ed). The Amsterdam Growth Study, a longitudinal analysis of health, fitness, and life-style. HK Sport Science Monograph series vol 6. Human Kinetics, Champaign, Ill, 1995

Kobayashi K, Kitamure M, Miura M. Aerobic power as related to body growth and training in Japanese boys: a longitudinal sutdy. J Appl. Physiol 44: 666-672, 1978

Koinzer K, Enderlein G, Herforth G. Untersuchungen zur Abhängigkeit der W170 vom Kalenderalter, vom biologischen entwicklungsstand und vom Ubungszustand bei 10- bis 14-järigen Jungen und Mädchen mittles dreifaktorieller Varianzanalyse. Medizin Sport 21: 201-206, 1981

Lanyon LE. The success and failure of the adaptive response to functional load-bearing in averting bone fracture. Bone 13: S17-S21, 1992

Lewis AB, Garu SM. Dental development by calcification stages from roentgenograms. The Angle Orthod 30: 70-77, 1960

Lohman TG. Advances in body composition assessment, Current Issues in Exercise Science Monograph nr 3 , Human Kinetics, Champaign, 1992

Marshall WA. Puberty. In: Falkner, Tanner, Human Growth vol 2: Postnatal growth: 141-181 (Plenum Press, New York, 1978)

Matkovic V, Fontana D, Tominac C, Goel P, Chesnut CH. Factors that influence peak bone mass formation: a study of calcium balance and the inheritance of bone mass in adolescent females. Am J Clin Nutr 52: 878-888, 1990

Meszaros J, Mohácsi J, Szabó S, Szmodis I. Assessment of biological development by anthropometric variables. In: Binkhorst, Kemper, Saris, Children and Exercise XI 15: 341-345, Human Kinetics, Champaign, 1985

Mirwald RL, Bailey DA, Cameron N, Rasmussen RL. Longitudinal comparison of aerobic power in active and inactive boys aged 7.0 to 17.0 years. Ann Hum Biol 8: 405-414, 1981

Post GB, Kemper HCG. Nutrient intake and biological maturation during adolescence. The Amsterdam growth and health longitudinal study. Eur J of Clin Nutrition 47: 400-408, 1993

Prader A. Biomedical and endocrinological aspects of normal growth and development: 1-23 (Plenum Press, New York, 1984)

Prahl-Andersen B, Roede MJ. The measurement of skeletal and dental maturity. In: Prahl-Andersen, Kowalski, Heydendael, A mixed-longitudinal interdisciplinary study of growth and development, vol 6: 491-521 (Academic Press, New York, 1979)

Recker RR, Davies KM, Hinders SM, Heaney RP, Stegman RP, Kimme DB. Bone gain in young adult women. JAMA 268: 2403-2408, 1992

Rico H, Revilla M, Hernandez ER, Vilaa LF, Alvarez del Buergo I. Sex differences in the acquisition of total bone mineral mass peak assessed through dual energy X-ray absorptiometry. Calcif Tissue Int 51: 251-254, 1992

Riis BJ, Krabbe S, Christianson C, Catherwood BD, Deftos LJ. Bone turnover in male puberty: a longitudinal study, N Eng J Med 316, 4: 174-178, 1985

Roche AF, Chumlea WC, Thissen D. Assessing the skeletal maturity of the hand-wrist: Fels Method. CC Thomas, Springfield Ill, 1988

Roche AF, Wainer H, Thissen D. Skeletal maturity: the knee joint as a biological indicator. Plenum, New York, 1975

Rubin CT, Lanyon LE. Regulation of bone formation by applied dynamic loads. J Bone and Joint Surg, 66A, 3: 397-402, 1884

Ruiz JC, Mandel C, Garabedian M. Influence of spontaneous calcium intake and physical exercise on the vertebral and femoral bone mineral density of children and adolescents. J Bone Min Res 10, 5: 675-682, 1995

Rutenfranz J, Lange Andersen K, Seliger V, Ilmarinen J, Klimmer F, Kylian H, Rutenfranz M, Ruppel M. Maximal aerobic power affected by maturation and body growth during childhood and adolescence. Eur J Pediat 139: 106-112, 1982

Sentipal JM, Wardlaw GM, Mahan J, Matkovic V. Influence of calcium intake and growth indexes on vertebral bone mineral density in young females. Am J Clin Nutr. 54: 425-428, 1991

Snow-Harter C, Marcus R. Exercise, bone mineral density, and osteoporosis. Exer Sport SCI Rev 19: 351-388, 1991

Southard RN, Morris JD, Mahan JD, Hayes JR, Torch MA, Sommer A. Bone mass in healthy children: Mesurement with quantitative DXA. Radiology 179: 735-738, 1991

Tanner JM. A history of the study of human growth. Cambridge University Press, London, 1981

Tanner JM, Whitehouse RH, Marshall WA, Healy MJR, Goldstein H. Assessment of skeletal maturity and prediction of adult height (TW2 method). Academic Press, London, 1975

Teegarden D, Proulx WR, Martin BR, Zhao J, Mccba GP, Lyle RM, Peacock M, Slemenda C, Johnston CC, Weaver CM. Peak bone mass in young women. J Bone Min Res, 10, 5: 711-715, 1995

Verschuur R. Daily physical activity and health; longitudinal changes during the teenage period De Vrieseborch, Haarlem, SO12, 1987

Weiner JS, Lourie JA. Human biology, a guide to field methods. IBP Handbook no 9. Blackwell, Oxford, 1969

Welten DC, Kemper HCG, Post GB, Staveren WA van. Meta-analysis of the effect of calcium intake on bone mass in young and middle aged females and males. J of Nutrition, nov, 1995

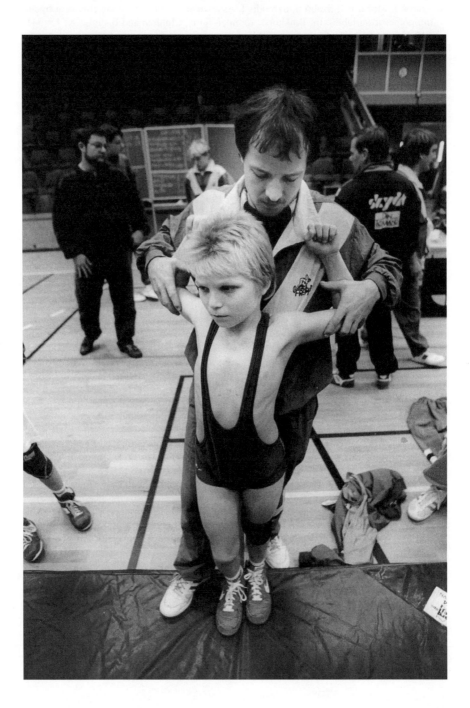

Chapter 11

Activity and Fitness of Youth: Are They Related? Do They Track?

Robert M. Malina

The physical activity and fitness of children and youth are issues of current interest among public health officials and many in the physical activity and sport sciences. As a rule, the current generation of children and youth is often characterized as either physically unfit or physically inactive, or both. The adequacy or inadequacy of current levels of activity and fitness, however, depend upon the criteria or reference used for comparison (Malina, 1995). In contrast, relatively little attention is given to the determinants of activity and fitness of children and youth.

Children and youth participate in a number of physical activities, which occur in a variety of forms and contexts, e.g., free movement, play, formal exercise, dance, physical education, sport, work, and probably others. In physiological terms, physical activity refers to "...bodily movement produced by skeletal muscles and resulting in energy expenditure (Bouchard et al., 1990, p. 6). The ability to perform physical activities requires some degree of proficiency in movement skills and physical fitness, and the value assigned to skill and fitness is dependent upon the cultural context. Physical activity and fitness thus have an essential cultural context. However, they cannot be approached from an exclusively biological or from an exclusively cultural (behavioral) perspective. A biocultural perspective is needed, and there is a need to understand the biocultural or biobehavioral determinants of activity and fitness.

Physical fitness of children and youth presently has a twofold context: motor and health-related fitness. The former is performance oriented and includes components of skilled movements, i.e., agility, balance, coordination, power, speed, strength and muscular endurance that enable the individual to perform a variety of physical activities. Health-related fitness, as the name implies, is oriented towards health status and is operationalized in terms of cardiorespiratory function, abdominal and low back musculoskeletal function, and fatness (Malina, 1991). In many developed countries, emphasis on the fitness of children and youth has shifted from a primary motor focus to a health-related focus over the past 15-20 years. The shift in emphasis to health-related fitness for children and youth is based on either one or both of the following premises related largely to adult health concerns: (1) regular physical activity during childhood and youth may function to prevent or impede the development of several adult diseases which include physical inactivity in a complex, multifactorial etiology: degenerative diseases of the heart and blood vessels, musculoskeletal disorders of the lower back, obesity and related complications; and (2) habits of regular physical activity during childhood and youth may directly and favorably influence physical activity habits in adulthood and in turn have a beneficial effect on the fitness and health status of adults (Malina, 1991). From the perspective of children and youth, the underlying assumptions of the health-related fitness paradigm are adult-driven, and the relevance of the health-related fitness paradigm to the health and fitness of children and youth can be questioned. The presently available evidence to support these assumptions, however, is not overwhelming (Malina, 1991, 1995), and the paradigm may be changing, i.e., from promotion of childhood activity and fitness that will lead to adult activity, fitness and health, to the development of a lifestyle pattern of physical activity that will carry over into the adult years (Rowland and Freedson, 1994). Presumably, the health benefits of activity may be related to the persistence of a regular pattern of physical activity.

Central to discussions of physical activity and fitness is the assumption that the two are related. Physical activity, of course, is a behavior, while physical fitness is to a large extent an adaptive state. Within this context, three questions are considered: (1) What is the relationship between activity and fitness - are the more active likely to be more fit?; (2) What is the relationship between fitness and activity - are the more fit likely to be more active?; (3) Is there a link between activity and fitness during childhood and youth and activity and fitness in adulthood?

Activity and fitness

It is generally assumed that the more habitually active are more fit, and that the relationship is causal. Corbin and Pangrazi (1993, p. 4), for example, state: "There is no doubt that regular physical activity builds physical fitness." Or more recently, Livingstone (1994, p. 207) states: "...physical activity and physical fitness are obviously related." The available data, however, do not support such a relationship in the general population of children and youth. In 6-9 year old children in second National Children and Youth Fitness Survey in the United States, for example, 28 indicators of physical activity, age and sex accounted for only 21% of the variance in the run-walk and 18% of the variance in fatness (Pate et al., 1990). A similar analysis relating habitual activity to the health-related fitness of 528 fourth grade children from southern California also resulted in low correlations. Estimated percentages of variance in fitness items accounted for by physical activity after controlling for sex were low, 3% to 11% (Sallis et al., 1993). Among Taiwanese youth 12-14 years of age, estimated daily energy expenditure and energy expenditure in moderate-to-vigorous physical activity was significantly related to the one-mile run and sit-and-reach, but was not related to sit-ups and the sum of skinfolds. Partial correlations controlling for age, sex, socioeconomic status and area of resident, though significant, were low, 0.12 to 0.19, and the amount of variance accounted for was <5% (Huang and Malina, in preparation). Among Quebec youth 9-18 years of age, canonical correlation analysis indicated only a weak association between estimated daily energy expenditure and energy expenditure in moderate-to-vigorous physical activity and several health-related fitness tests. The variance shared by the canonical variates ranged from 11% to 21% (Malina et al., 1996). Hence, the relationship between habitual physical activity and the health-related fitness of children, though statistically significant, is not strong. Studies of other samples of adolescents give similar results (Aaron et al., 1993; Renson et al., 1990; Watson and O'Donovan, 1977). The general pattern of results from correlational studies, using a variety of indicators of physical activity and health-related fitness, indicate a significant but relatively weak relationship between activity and fitness, and suggest that factors other than physical activity exert more influence on the health-related fitness of children and youth.

The preceding evaluates the relationship between physical activity and various components of health-related fitness, and does not consider the effects of specific activity programs, or training at various intensities, on indicators of fitness. Experimental studies of the effects of systematic training and/or physical activity on health-related fitness during childhood and adolescence generally indicate improvements in specific components (Pate and Ward, 1990; Rowland, 1985; Sale, 1989; Vogel, 1986). With few exceptions, the studies are short term and ordinarily do not include a follow-up component. The studies are seemingly more focused on the effects of training per se, i.e., trainability, and not on the persistence of the beneficial responses. The question of interest should perhaps be: How much activity is necessary to develop and maintain high levels of fitness in children and youth? Or, what is the healthy level of physical activity for children and youth?

Active and inactive youth

It is possible that the relationship between activity and fitness is masked by the broad range of variability in heterogenous samples of children and youth and is perhaps more apparent in comparisons of groups at the extremes of the physical activity continuum. Active and inactive 10-12 year old United States youth in the first phase of the National Children and Youth Fitness Survey did not differ in the one mile run, while active 13-15 year old active youth performed better; at older ages, only active boys 16+ years performed better in the one mile run, while active and inactive girls of the same age did not differ (Blair et al., 1989). Among Taiwanese youth 12-14 years of age, those in the highest quartile of estimated energy expenditure had significantly better one mile run times and sit and reach scores than those in the lowest quartile. In contrast, boys and girls in the highest and lowest quartiles of estimated energy expenditure did not differ in sit-ups and sum of skinfolds (Huang and Malina, in preparation). The cross-sectional observations are reasonably consistent with longitudinal data on the health-related fitness of active and inactive adolescents. In the Saskatchewan Growth Study (Mirwald et al., 1981; Mirwald and Bailey, 1986), inactive boys had lower absolute and relative VO2max than active boys and those with average levels of activity from 8-16 years, while the active boys had a greater relative VO2max than normally active and inactive boys before, during and after the adolescent growth spurt. In the Leuven Growth Study of Belgian Boys (Beunen et al., 1992), active boys performed better than inactive boys only in the pulse rate recovery after a step test and the flexed arm hang (functional strength) from 13-18 years. The two groups did not differ in leg lifts (abdominal strength), sit and reach (flexiblity), and four skinfolds. In the Amsterdam Growth and Health Study (Verschuur, 1987), active boys 13-16 years performed better than inactive boys in maximal aerobic power, the 12 minute run, and functional strength, while active girls performed better in maximal aerobic power and the 12 minute run. In contrast, active and inactive boys and girls, respectively, did not differ in the sit and reach. Although methods of assessment and criteria for active and inactive youth vary among studies, and although data are more available for males, one consistent observation surfaces in both cross-sectional and longitudinal studies - more active youth are more fit in cardiovascular endurance tasks. In contrast, results for other components of health-related fitness, i.e., lower back flexibility, abdominal strength and fatness, are inconsistent.

Fit and unfit youth

The preceding is based on the assumption that habitual physical activity is related to fitness, and the available data suggest that being active does not neccessarily guarantee better fitness. Comparisons of the habitual physical activity of fit and unfit children and youth may help clarify the situation, but such data are not presently extensive. Are the more fit in fact more active? This question was addressed in Taiwanese youth 12-14 years of age (Huang and Malina, in preparation). The subjects were classified as fit (highest quartile) or unfit (lowest quartile) for the four components of the AAHPERD health-related fitness test. Note, the position of the quartiles was inverted for the one mile run and sum of skinfolds because a lower score indicates better fitness. Boys and girls classified as fit in the one mile run and the sit and reach had a significantly greater estimated daily energy expenditure (kcal x kg^{-1} x day^{-1}) than those classified as unfit. In contrast, boys and girls classified as fit and unfit in sit-ups and sum of skinfolds did not differ in estimated energy expenditure. The activity status of fit and unfit youth in each health-related fitness was rather heterogeneous. For example, among the 34 boys classified as fit in the one mile run, 15 were active (highest quartile for estimated energy expenditure) and 7 were inactive (lowest quartile for estimated energy expenditure). In contrast, among the 34 boys classified as unfit in the one mile run, 3 were active and 16 were inactive. Results were generally similar for girls. Among the 36 girls classified as fit in the one mile run, 16 were active and 8 were inactive, while among the 36 girls classified as unfit in the one mile run, 5 were active and 13 were inactive. The activity status of youth classified as fit and unfit in the other health-related fitness tests also showed considerable overlap. Thus, although youth classified as fit in some health-related fitness items are, on average, more active, there is much variability. These results echo the earlier observations of Lange Anderson et al. (1984, p. 435) in a study of 14-18 year old boys and girls using annual sport activity scores as an indicator of habitual physical activity and maximal aerobic power as the index of fitness: "...among those with the poorest fitness, there are sedentary, moderately active and very active children. Similarly, there are sedentary, moderately active and very active children among those who are in excellent physical condition."

Overview of activity-fitness relationships

Although physical activity and health-related physical fitness are significantly correlated, the relationship is not strong, and indicators of actvity account for a relatively small percentage of the variation in several indicators of fitness. Several factors probably contribute to these observations in children and youth. The results reflect, in part, the measures or estimates of habitual physical activity, and the measures of fitness. They are imperfect at best. Children's levels of physical activity do not ordinarily, or regularly, reach aerobic levels. Hence, why should a strong relationship between aerobic fitness (VO_2max) and physical activity be expected? On the other hand, is VO_2max the best measure of fitness, or is it a laboratory measure aimed at a reference for comparison? The field measures of fitness reflect the operational definition of health-related fitness, which may need modification. What is the relative importance of the health-related fitness tests to the short- and long-term health status of children and youth?

Growth (increase in size) and maturation (tempo and timing of progress towards the mature state) per se are also factors affecting the relationship, or lack of relationship, between activity and fitness. Components of fitness change with normal growth and maturation independent of physical activity (Malina and Bouchard, 1991). Hence, it is often difficult to partition effects to activity from those due to growth and maturation. What are the specific contributions of growth and maturation to fitness and perhaps activity? How much of the variance in physical fitness items can be attributed to variation in maturity status? Such a question is confounded in part by the fact that indicators of maturity status are related to chronological age and body size, which in turn are related to physical fitness. Among Belgian adolescent boys, for example, the interaction of skeletal age (indicator of biological maturation) and chronological age, or in combination with height and/or weight, had the highest predictive value for a variety of fitness components. The explained variance reached 33% to 56% for several strength items (Beunen et al., 1981). On the other hand, skeletal age did not have the same predictive value for the fitness of Belgian girls. Interactions of chronological age and weight, or height and weight had the highest predictive value for a variety of fitness tests, and these interactions accounted for a smaller percentage of the variance than in boys (Beunen et al., 1996). Thus, in these two studies of Belgian youth, skeletal age is a more important predictor of fitness in boys than in girls.

Childhood-adolescence-adulthood:
A continuum

The promotion of physical activity and health-related fitness of children and youth is based in part on the assumption that a physically active lifestyle developed during the growing years will carry over into adulthood. Simons-Morton et al. (1988, p. 404), for example, explicitly state: "Adulthood physical activity is strongly influenced by dispositions and habits established early in life...," while Meredith and Dwyer (1991, p. 313) note: "Activity patterns developed during these years (adolescence) carry over to later life and affect morbidity and mortality." More recently, Livingstone (1994, p. 207) offers the following: "Physical activity is accepted as one of the major prerequisites for normal growth and development of children and adolescents. Other desired outcomes include psychological well-being and the potential development of positive attitudes and habits as a foundation for an active lifestyle in adulthood." What evidence supports these generalizations? How well does activity or fitness during childhood and youth track into adulthood?

Correlations between indicators of physical activity during adolescence and activity in adulthood tend to be low, ranging from 0.05 to 0.39 (Andersen and Haraldsdottir, 1993; Vanreusel et al., 1993a, 1993b; van Mechelen and Kemper, 1995). Correlations across various age spans in adulthood are only slightly higher, 0.23 to 0.48 (Lee et al., 1992; Vanreusel et al., 1993b; van Mechelen and Kemper, 1995). Various measures of health-related fitness, e.g., aerobic power, strength, flexibility, and fatness track significantly across childhood and adolescence, but interage correlations are generally low and at best moderate (Malina, 1990a, 1990b). Data are less extensive from adolescence into adulthood. Among Danish subjects, interage correlations between 15-19 years and 23-27 years for absolute (L x min^{-1}) and relative (ml x min^{-1} x kg^{-1}) VO$_2$max were 0.51 and 0.35, respectively, in males and 0.72 and 0.48, respectively, in females, while corresponding correlations for estimated relative fatness were 0.72 and 0.46 in males and females, respectively (Andersen and Haraldsdottir, 1993). Interage correlations for indicators of health-related fitness in 173 Belgian males followed from 13-18 years and then tested at 30 years of age were better from late adolescence (18-30 years) than from early adolescence (13-30 years) into adulthood (Beunen et al., 1992). Among health-related fitness items, flexibility of the lower back tracked reasonably well into early adulthood (0.68 to 0.82), measures of subcutaneous fatness and muscular strength and endurance tracked moderately (0.35 to 0.60), while heart rate recovery after a step test tracked poorly (0.26 to 0.40).

Other studies utilize different estimates of activity during youth and in adulthood. For example, British youth of both sexes rated by their teachers as above average in sport at 13 years of age and as energetic at 15 years of age were one and one-half times more likely to participate in active leisure pursuites at 36 years of age (Kuh and Cooper, 1992). Swedish youth of both sexes who had more prior experiences with sport and physical activity at 15 years of age (defined as a high grade in physical education in 8th grade, 4+ hrs x wk^{-1} practice of sport in a club and sport club membership), had a higher readiness for physical activity at 30 years of age, males more so than females. And, individuals with higher psychological readiness (defined as a more positive view of the body and capabilities in sport) tended to be more active at 30 years of age (Engstrom, 1986, 1991).

A related question is the association, if any, between fitness during childhood and youth and adult involvement in physical activity. Physically active young adult American males 23-25 years of age had better motor fitness scores (AAHPERD Fitness Test) as 10-11 and 15-18 years of age than inactive young adult males (Dennison et al., 1988). Boys whose performances on the 600 yard run were below the 20th percentile were at a greater risk for adult physical inactivity. In Swedish adults 27 years of age, aerobic capacity at 16 years of age accounted for about 31%

and 24% of the variation in leisure time physical activity at 27 years of age in women and men, respectively. Further, physical activity, grades in physical education and strength at 16 years of age added to the predictability of activity at 27 years of age women, but not in men (Glenmark et al., 1994). In a study comparing leisure patterns during adolescence and 37 years later, bivariate correlations between adolescent and adult participation in sports were low, 0.13 in males and 0.25 in females. However, in a multivariate context, adolescent sport participation had a greater effect on adult sport participation in women than in men (Scott and Willits, 1989).

Implications

Physical activity and health-related physical fitness are significantly correlated in children and youth, but the relationship is not strong. This suggests that other factors are important determinants of levels of habitual physical activity and fitness. Quite often, however, children and youth are labeled as inactive and unfit, and school physical education programs are implicated as a major etiological agent. Specifically, the physical education profession is criticized for placing too much emphasis on sports skills. Moreover, many involved in public health or the health promotion field hold that cardiorespiratory endurance and fitness should be the objective of physical education at all grade levels, particularly in the context of the goals of the Healthy People 2000 (U.S. Public Health Service, 1990). The objectives emphasize cardiorespiratory fitness as a major health-related objective for children and youth; for example: "Increase ... to at least 75% the proportion of children and adolescents aged 6 through 17 years who engage in vigorous physical activity that promotes the development and maintenance of cardiorespiratory fitness; 3 or more days per week 20 minutes or more per occasion" (U.S. Public Health Service, 1990, p. 92]. In keeping with this focus, Simons-Morton et al. (1988, pp. 419-422) suggest that

> "Current practices in PE are not consistent with health and fitness goals. What is needed is a major change in the philosophy and practice of PE from the current emphasis on motor skills and sports, to an emphasis on physical fitness education. ... Especially in elementary school, children should spend nearly every minute during PE in enjoyable MVPA (moderate to vigorous physical activity). We recommend that school districts implement cardiovascular fitness-oriented physical education and health-related fitness testing, and evaluate PE on the basis of how much MVPA children obtain during PE."

Subsequently, Simons-Morton et al. (1993, p. 264) emphasize that

> "Health promotion is the contemporary rationale for physical education, and the health of children is best served by physical education programs that provide substantial amounts of moderate to vigorous physical activity and promote out-of-school lifetime physical activity."

More recently, Livingstone (1994, p. 218) stresses that

> "...the current emphasis on motor skills and sports in physical education classes is unlikely to foster the physical, psychological and social events which combine to promote the concept of total fitness. ... By shifting the emphasis to increased participation in enjoyable and stimulating MVPA, children are more likely to want to keep participating for its own sake."

The preceding views are critical of physical education as it is presently taught, motor skills, and sports. These views overlook the importance of context, i.e., the context of physical activity. Children and youth, and probably many adults, do not exercise for the sake of exercise! Further, the motivation for activity is probably different for children and youth. They characteristically view activity in the context of fun and social relationships, i.e., enjoyment and to be with friends. Children and youth do not ordinarily think in terms of short- and/or long-term health status. What is the most common context of physical activity for children and youth? Physical activity occurs most often in the context of games and sport, all of which include a motor skill component, and enjoyment and success are often related to skill. I would suggest that a major hurdle to the promotion of physical activity is not school physical education and its emphasis on motor skills and sports; rather, it is the emphasis on highly organized and specialized sport for children and youth which favors the allocation of resources, facilities and other services to the elite with a corresponding lack for the general population of children and youth.

Discussions of physical activity and health-related fitness in children and youth also include the assumption that a physically active lifestyle and/or fitness developed during the growing years will carry over into adulthood. Relationships between childhood and adolescent activity and fitness and adult physical activity are suggestive but weak. However, several trends merit closer attention. First, the data are limited largely to males, emphasizing the need for further study of childhood and adolescent correlates of adult activity and fitness in women. There may be sex differences. Glenmark et al. (1994), for example, showed that a combination of physical characteristics, performance and activity at 16 years of age explained more of the variation in leisure time physical activity at 27 years of age in women (82%) than in men (47%). Second, it appears that those who are more active in sport during childhood and adolescence are more likely to be active as adults. Third, those who are less fit during childhood and adolescence are at greater risk to be inactive as young adults. Fourth, data on the transitional years from the late teenages into adulthood are lacking. This is a period of major change in lifestyle which has implications for activity and fitness (Malina, 1990, 1994). Fifth, data on the relationship, if any, between a physically active, fit lifestyle during childhood and adolescence and adult health and risk of mortality are lacking. Adult health status and risk of mortality are apparently more related to current level of physical activity rather than activity in the past (Fox and Skinner, 1964; Paffenbarger et al., 1986). One component of health-related fitness, however, is important. Evidence suggests that overweight during childhood and adolescence is associated with long term morbidity and mortality 30 to 55 years later (Must et al., 1992; Nieto et al., 1992).

Recommendations

The physical activity and physical fitness of children and youth need to be viewed in a context broader than that implied in the concept of health-related fitness, and more specifically, cardiovascular fitness. Physical activity and fitness are biocultural processes. There is a need to understand the biocultural determinants of activity and fitness not only among children and youth, but through the lifespan. Variability is a fact of nature. Not all individuals are equally skilled or active, and not all individuals need the same amount or intensity of physical activity.

Children and youth are not miniature adults. They have many needs and tasks related to physical growth and maturation and to the development of behavioral competence in a variety of domains. The processes of growth, maturation and development are interrelated, and should not be viewed independently. Physical activity and fitness are integral parts of growth, maturation and development and should be reinstated into the context of childhood and adolescence. In other words, what is the role of physical activity and fitness for children and youth as children and youth, and not when they will be adults?

Motor and health-related fitness are not mutually exclusive, and physical education is more than moderate to vigorous physical activity and cardiovascular fitness. A balance is essential in the context of the developmental needs and tasks of children and youth. A foundation of competence in motor skills is a necessary requisite for subsequent enjoyment of physical activity.

References

Aaron DJ, Kriska AM, Dearwater SR, Anderson RL, OLsen TL, Cauley JA, Laporte RE: The epidemiology of leisure physical activity in an adolescent population. Med Sci Sports Exerc 1993; 25:847-853.

Andersen LB, Haraldsdottir J: Tracking of cardiovascular disease risk factors including maximal oxygen uptake and physical activity from late teenage to adulthood: An 8-year follow-up study. J Intern Med 1993; 234:309-315.

Beunen G, Lefevre J, Claessens AL, Lysens R, Maes H, Renson R, Simons J, Vanden Eynde B, Vanreusel B, Van Den Bossche C: Age-specific correlation analysis of longitudinal physical fitness levels in men. Eur J Appl Physiol 1992; 64:538-545.

Beunen GP, Malina RM, Lefevre J, Claessens AL, Renson R, Vanden Eynde B, Vanreusel B, Simons J: Skeletal maturation, somatic growth, and physical fitness in girls 6-16 years of age. 1996; submitted for publication.

Beunen GP, Malina RM, Renson R, Simons J, Ostyn M, Lefevre J: Physical activity and growth, maturation and performance: A longitudinal study. Med Sci Sports Exerc 1992; 24:576-585.

Beunen G, Ostyn M, Simons J, Renson R, Van Gerven D: Chronological age and biological age as related to physical fitness in boys 12 to 19 years. Ann Hum Biol 1981; 8:321-331.

Blair SN, Clark DG, Cureton KJ, Powell KE: Exercise and fitness in childhood: Implications for a lifetime of health. In Gisolfi CV, Lamb DR, eds. Perspectives in exercise science and sports medicine. Volume 2. Youth, Exercise and Sport. Indianpolis: Benchmark Press; 1989:401-430.

Bouchard C, Shephard RJ, Stephens T, Sutton JR, McPherson BD, eds. Exercise, fitness, and health: The consensus statement. In: Bouchard C, Shephard RJ, Stephens T, Sutton JR, McPherson BD, eds. Exercise, fitness, and health: A consensus of current knowledge. Champaign, IL: Human Kinetics; 1990:3-28.

Corbin CB, Pangrazi RP: The health benefits of physical activity. Phys Act Fit Res Digest 1993; 1:1-7 (Feb).

Dennison BA, Straus AH, Mellits ED, Charney E: Childhood physical fitness tests: Predictor of adult physical activity levels? Pediatrics 1988; 82:324-330.

Engstrom LM, The process of socialization into keep-fit activities. J Sports Sci 1986; 8:89-97.

Engstrom LM: Exercise adherence in sport for all from youth to adulthood. In: Oja P, Telama R, eds. Sport for all. Amsterdam: Elsevier Science, 1991:473-483.

Fox SM, Skinner JM: Physical activity and cardiovascular health. Am J Cardiol 1964; 14:731-746.

Glenmark B, Hedberg G, Jansson E: Prediction of physical activity level in adulthood by physical characteristics, physical performance and physical activity in adolescence: An 11-year follow-up study. Eur J Appl Physiol 1994; 69: 530-538.

Huang YC, Malina RM: Physical activity and health-related physical fitness in Taiwanese youth 12-14 years of age, in preparation.

Kuh DJL, Cooper C: Physical activity at 36 years: Patterns and childhood predictors in a longitudinal study. J Epidemiol Comm Health 1992; 46:114-119.

Lange Andersen K, Ilmarinen J, Rutenfranz J, Ottmann W, Berndt I, Kylian H, Ruppel M: Leisure time sport activities and maximal aerobic power during late adolescence. Eur J Appl Physiol 1984; 52:431-436.

Lee IM, Paffenbarger RS Jr, Hsieh CC: Time trends in physical activity among college alumni, 1962-1988. Am J Epidemiol 1992; 135:915-925.

Livingstone MBE: Energy expenditure and physical activity in relation to fitness in children. Proc Nutr Soc 1994; 53:207-221.

Malina RM: Growth, exercise, fitness, and later outcomes. In Bouchard C, Shephard RJ, Stephens T, Sutton JR, McPherson BD, eds. Exercise, fitness, and health: A consensus of current knowledge. Champaign, IL: Human Kinetics, 1990a:637-653.

Malina RM: Tracking of physical fitness and performance during growth. In: Beunen G, Ghesquiere J, Reybrouck T, Claessens AL, eds. Children and exercise. Stuttgart: Ferdinand Enke Verlag, 1990b:1-10.

Malina RM: Fitness and performance: Adult health and the culture of youth. In: Park RJ, Eckert HM, eds. New possibilities, new paradigms? (American Academy of Physical Education Papers No. 24). Champaign, IL: Human Kinetics; 1991:30-38.

Malina RM: Physical activity: Relationship to growth, maturation, and physical fitness. In: Bouchard C, Shephard RJ, Stephens T, eds. Physical activity, fitness, and health. Champaign, IL: Human Kinetics; 1994:918-930.

Malina RM: Physical activity and fitness of children and youth: Questions and implications. Med Exerc Nutr Health 1995; 5:125-137.

Malina RM, Bouchard C: Growth, maturation, and physical activity. Champaign, IL: Human Kinetics; 1991.

Malina RM, Katzmarzyk PT, Song TMK, Bouchard C: A multivariate analysis of physical activity and fitness in school-aged children and youth. Am J Hum Biol 1996; 8, in press (abstract).

Meredith CN, Dwyer JT: Nutrition and exercise: Effects on adolescent health. Ann Rev Publ Health 1991; 12:309-333.

Mirwald RL, Bailey DA, Cameron N, Rasmussen RL: Longitudinal comparison of aerobic power in active and inactive boys 7.0 to 17.0 years. Ann Human Biol 1981; 8:405-414.

Mirwald RL, Bailey DA: Maximal aerobic power. London, Ontario: Sports Dynamics; 1986.

Must A, Jacques PF, Dallal GE, Bajema CJ, Dietz WH, Long-term morbidity and mortality of overweight adolescents. N Engl J Med 1992; 327:1350-1355.

Nieto FJ, Szklo M, Comstock GW: Childhood weight and growth rate as predictors of adult mortality. Am J Epidemiol 1992; 136:201-213.

Paffenbarger RS Jr, Hyde RT, Wing AL, Hsieh CC: Physical activity, all-cause mortality, and longevity of college alumni. New Eng J Med 1986; 314:605-613.

Pate RR, Dowda M, Ross JG: Associations between physical activity and physical fitness in American children. Am J Dis Child 1990; 144:1123-1129.

Pate RR, Ward DS: Endurance exercise trainability in children and youth. Adv Sports Med Fitness 1990; 3:37-55.

Renson R, Beunen G, Claessens AL, Colla R, Lefevre J, Ostyn M, Schueremans C, Simons J, Taks M, Van Gerven D, Vanreusel B: Physical fitness variation among 13 to 18 year old boys and girls according to sport participation. In: Beunen G, Ghesquiere J, Reybrouck T, Claessens AL, eds. Children and exercise. Stuttgart: Ferdinand Enke Verlag; 1990: 136-144.

Rowland TW: Aerobic response to endurance training in prepubescent children: A critical analysis. Med Sci Sports Exerc 1985; 17:493-497.

Rowland TW, Freedson PS: Physical activity, fitness, and health in children: A close look. Pediatrics 1994; 93:669-672.

Sale DG: Strength training in children. In: Gisolfi CV, Lamb DR, eds. Perspectives in exercise science and sports medicine. Volume 2. Youth, exercise, and sport. Indianpolis: Benchmark Press; 1989:165-216.

Sallis JF, McKenzie TL, Alcaraz JE: Habitual physical activity and health-related physical fitness in fourth-grade children. Am J Dis Child 1993; 147:890-896.

Scott D, Willits FK: Adolescent and adult leisure patterns: A 37-year follow-up study. Leisure Sciences 1989; 11:323-335.

Simons-Morton BG, Parcel GS, O'Hara NM, Blair SN, Pate RR: Health-related physical fitness in childhood: Status and recommendations. Ann Rev Publ Health 1988; 9:403-425.

Simons-Morton BG, Taylor WC, Snider SA, Huang IW: The physical activity of fifth-grade students during physical education classes. Am J Publ Health 1993; 83:262-264.

U.S. Public Health Service: Healthy people 2000: National health promotion and disease prevention objectives. Washington, DC: U.S. Government Printing Office; 1990.

van Mechelen W, Hemper HCG: Habitual physical activity in longitudinal perspective. In: HCG Kemper, ed. The Amsterdam Growth Study: A longitudinal analysis of health, fitness, and lifestyle. Champaign, IL: Human Kinetics, 1995:135-158.

Vanreusel B, Renson R, Beunen G, Claessens A, Lefevre J, Lysens R, Maes H, Simons J, Vanden Eynde B: Adherence to sport from youth to adulthood: A longitudinal study on socialization. In: Duquet W, De Knop P, Bollaert L, eds. Youth sport: A social approach. Brussels: VUB Press, 1993a:99-109.

Vanreusel B, Renson R, Beunen G, Claessens A, Lefevre J, Lysens R, Maes H, Simons J, Vanden Eynde B: Involvement in physical activity from youth to adulthood: A longitudinal analysis. In: Claessens AL, Lefevre J, Vanden Eynde B, eds. World-wide variation in physical fitness. Leuven: Institute of Physical Education, Katholieke Universiteit Leuven, 1993b:187-195.

Verschuur R: Daily physical activity: Longitudinal changes during the teenage period. Haarlem, The Netherlands: Uitgeverij de Vrieseborch; 1987.

Vogel PG: Effects of physical education programs on children. In: Seefeldt V, ed. Physical activity and well-being. Reston, VA: American Alliance for Health, Physical Education, Recreation and Dance; 1986:455-509.

Watson AWS, O'Donovan DJ: The relationship of level of habitual physical activity to measures of leanness-fatness, physical working capacity, strength, and motor ability in 17 and 18 year old males. Eur J Appl Physiol 1977; 37:93-100.

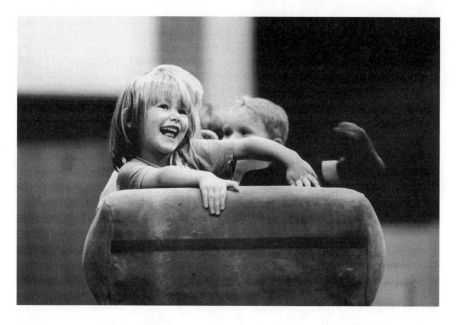

Chapter 12

The Assessment and Interpretation of Aerobic Fitness in Children and Adolescents: An Update

Neil Amstrong and Joanne Welsman

This paper presents data collected in our laboratory to develop further our recent review of the assessment and interpretation of aerobic fitness in children and adolescents (Armstrong and Welsman, 1994). It will focus specifically on whether peak oxygen uptake (peak $\dot{V}O_2$) can be regarded as a maximal index of young people's aerobic fitness and it will address the problem of interpreting growth-related changes in peak $\dot{V}O_2$.

Is peak $\dot{V}O_2$ a maximal index of children and adolescents' aerobic fitness?

Maximal oxygen uptake ($\dot{V}O_2$ max), the highest rate at which an individual can consume oxygen during exercise, limits the capacity to perform aerobic exercise and is therefore widely recognised as the best single indicator of aerobic fitness (Åstrand and Rodahl, 1986). The conventional model assumes that $\dot{V}O_2$ rises with increasing exercise intensity up to a point beyond which no fufther increase in $\dot{V}O_2$ takes place, even though the subject is still able to increase his/her exercise intensity. Exercise beyond the point of levelling of oxygen consumption (a $\dot{V}O_2$ plateau) is apparently supported exclusively by anaerobic energy sources resulting in an intracellular assimilation of lactate, acidosis and inevitably termination of the exercise. An absolute levelling of $\dot{V}O_2$ with increasing exercise intensity is, however, seldom seen and a number of less rigorous criteria of a $\dot{V}O_2$ plateau have been proposed. These include a rise in $\dot{V}O_2$ during the final exercise period of 150 ml x min[-1], $\leq 5\%$ or ≤ 2 ml x kg[-1] x min[-1]. Both methodological (Myers et al., 1989, 1990) and theoretical (Noakes, 1988) bases of the $\dot{V}O_2$ plateau phenomenon have been challenged but it is still used as the principal criterion for establishing $\dot{V}O_2$ max during a laboratory exercise test (Åstrand and Rodahl, 1986; Thoden, 1991).

Åstrand (1952), in his classical study of physical work capacity in relation to age and sex, observed that only 50% of subjects aged 6 to 17 years demonstrated a

$\dot{V}O_2$ plateau. Subsequent studies have reported that only a minority of children and adolescents demonstrate a plateau in $\dot{V}O_2$ during either treadmill or cycle ergometer exercise (collated by Rowland and Cunningham, 1992; Rivera-Brown et al., 1992). The appropriate term to use with young people is therefore peak $\dot{V}O_2$, which represents the highest oxygen uptake elicited during an exercise test to voluntary exhaustion, rather than $\dot{V}O_2$ max, which conventionally implies the existence of a $\dot{V}O_2$ plateau.

Table 1: Peak physiologic data of boys who showed a plateau and no plateau in oxygen consumption

Status	Group	n	peak $\dot{V}O_2$ ($l \times min^{-1}$)	peak heart rate ($b \times min^{-1}$)	peak blood lactate ($mmol \times l^{-1}$)
Pubescent:	No Plateau	80	2.34 ± 0.62	200 ± 8	5.2 ± 1.7
	Plateau	33	2.24 ± 0.57	202 ± 9	5.5 ± 2.2
Prepubescent	No Plateau	84	1.81 ± 0.24	200 ± 7	4.7 ± 1.4
	Plateau	27	1.72 ± 0.27	199 ± 7	4.4 ± 1.4

Exercise tests with children and adolescents are usually terminated when the young person, despite strong verbal encouragement from the experimenters, is unwilling or unable to continue. The experimenters are then left with the problem of deciding whether the youngster has delivered a maximal effort. We believe that habituation to the laboratory environment, subjective criteria of intense effort (e.g. hyperpnea, facial flushing, sweating, unsteady gait) and the paediatric exercise testing experience of the experimenters are vital ingredients in making this decision as no single variable can confirm a maximal effort. Nevertheless, despite wide individual variability we find peak heart rate and peak respiratory exchange ratio (RER) valuable subsidiary criteria when using a progressive, incremental test. Some laboratories recommend high postexercise blood lactate levels (e.g. 6-7 mmol x l^{-1}) as a subsidiary criterion of maximal exercise (Cumming et al., 1980; Krahenbuhl et al., 1985) but we have found peak blood lactates problematic, particularly with young children (Armstrong and Welsman, 1994; Welsman and Armstrong, in press). In our experience young people can exercise to exhaustion without generating high levels of blood lactate. As it is advisable to encourage children and adolescents to cool down with exercise of gradually reducing intensity following maximal exertion, we take capillary blood samples immediately exercise terminates and use a whole blood assay (Williams et al., 1992). With this technique we have reported mean blood lactates at peak $\dot{V}O_2$ of 5.4 ± 1.7 mmol x l^{-1} and 6.1 ± 1.7 mmol x l^{-1} with 11 to 16 year old boys (n=96) and girls (n=91) respectively (Williams and Armstrong, 1991) and 4.7 ± 1.4 mmol x l^{-1} and 5.1 ± 1.9 mmol x l^{-1} with prepubescent boys (n=111) and girls (n=53) respectively (Armstrong et al., in press). Interestingly, we have been unable to identify significant changes in blood lactate at peak $\dot{V}O_2$ with measures of maturity (Williams and Armstrong, 1991; Welsman et al., 1994).

It has been suggested that better test-retest reliability can be achieved when a $\dot{V}O_2$ plateau criterion is used (Freedson and Goodman, 1993) but this remains to be proven (Krahenbuhl et al., 1985). Some authors have argued that the failure to demonstrate a $\dot{V}O_2$ plateau may be related to low levels of motivation or low anaerobic capacity (Cunningham et al., 1977; Krahenbuhl et al., 1985; Rowland, 1993). However, recent data from our laboratory have shown that although only a minority of both adolescents (Armstrong et al., 1991) and prepubescent children (Armstrong et al., in press) may exhibit a $\dot{V}O_2$ plateau those who plateau do not have higher peak $\dot{V}O_2$, heart rate or blood lactate than those not demonstrating a $\dot{V}O_2$ plateau. (see tables 1 and 2)

Table 2: Peak physiologic data of girls who showed a plateau and no plateau in oxygen consumption

Status	Group	n	peak $\dot{V}O_2$ (lx min^{-1})	peak heart rate b x min^{-1})	peak blood lactate mmol x l^{-1})
Pubescent:	No Plateau	65	1.93 ± 0.40	201 ± 8	6.1 ± 1.8
	Plateau	39	1.86 ± 0.30	203 ± 8	5.9 ± 1.7
Prepubescent	No Plateau	34	1.49 ± 0.26	202 ± 7	5.0 ± 2.0
	Plateau	19	1.41 ± 0.14	201 ± 7	5.3 ± 1.9

In a recent study (Armstrong et al., under review) we determined the peak $\dot{V}O_2$ of 20 boys and 20 girls (mean age 9.9 ± 0.4 y) using a discontinuous, incremental test in which, following a warm-up, the treadmill speed was held constant at 1.94 m x s^{-1} and the gradient was raised by 2.5% every 3 min until voluntary exhaustion. One week later the children returned to the laboratory and following a 3 min warm-up the treadmill speed was increased to 1 . 94 m x s^{-1} and the gradient raised to 2.5% greater than that which had produced an exhaustive effort on the first test. The child ran to exhaustion. A third test was conducted similarly one week later but the treadmill gradient was raised to 5% greater than that which had produced an exhaustive effort on the first test. The data were accepted if the child ran for at least 2 min at supramaximal exercise intensity.

Eighteen girls and 17 boys completed all three exercise tests. Using ≤ 2 ml x kg^{-1} x min^{-1} increase in $\dot{V}O_2$ as the criterion 7 (39%) girls and 6 (35%) boys demonstrated a $\dot{V}O_2$ plateau. In accord with our earlier reports (Armstrong et al., 1991; Armstrong et al., in press) there were no significant differences in either anthropometrical or peak physiologic data between those who demonstrated a $\dot{V}O_2$ plateau and those who did not exhibit a $\dot{V}O_2$ plateau. Fufthermore, no significant differences in peak $\dot{V}O_2$ were identified between the three tests in either sex. With both boys and girls tests two and three elicited significantly higher peak RER, peak blood lactate and peak ventilation than test one. In other words, despite an increased anaerobic contribution to the exercise supramaximal exercise failed to induce an increase in the peak $\dot{V}O_2$ determined during a progressive, incremental test.

These findings concur with those of Rowland (1993) and strongly support the premise that a $\dot{V}O_2$ plateau should not be used as a requirement for defining a maximal exercise test with children. The mean blood lactates at peak $\dot{V}O_2$ in test one were 6.4 ± 1.3 mmol x l⁻¹ in girls and 5.7 ± 1.7 mmol x l⁻¹ in boys and rose to 8.3 ± 2.1 mmol x l⁻¹ and 9.3 ± 1.9 mmol x l⁻¹ respectively in test three. These data confirm our view that children can exercise to exhaustion without generating high levels of blood lactate and suggest that a requirement for high post exercise blood lactate levels as a criterion of maximal aerobic exercise (peak $\dot{V}O_2$) is untenable.

In summary, the requirement of a $\dot{V}O_2$ plateau before peak $\dot{V}O_2$ can be regarded as a maximal index of aerobic fitness is not tenable. Peak heart rate and RER are useful objective criteria that experimenters can use to support subjective observations when deciding whether the child or adolescent has demonstrated a maximal effort. The use of blood lactate measures, especially with young children, are problematic and some children can achieve peak $\dot{V}O_2$ without generating high levels of blood lactate.

Interpreting growth-related changes in aerobic fitness

In several recent publications ourselves and others have confirmed Tanner's (1949) concerns with the use of per body mass ratios (ratio standards) to partition out body size differences from measures of performance including peak aerobic and anaerobic function. The use of ratio standards has obscured sex, age and maturational differences identifiable when data are normalised using alternative statistical models (Eston et al., 1991; Winter et al., 1991, 1992; Nevill et al., 1992; Williams et al., 1992; Welsman et al., in press).

Several studies have employed linear regression scaling models (Tanner, 1949; Williams et al., 1992; Toth et al., 1993, Winter et al., 1991) and their widespread adoption as a data normalisation technique has been strongly recommended (Toth et al., 1993). However, such an emphatic recommendation may be misplaced (Cooper and Berman, 1995). The caveats associated with linear modelling are well-documented (Nevill et al., 1992, Winter, 1992) and there are situations where linear adjustment models (regression standards) do not provide an adequate statistical fit for performance data despite a reduction in the residual error as compared with a ratio scaling model (Nevill et al., 1992; Welsman et al., in press). Here, nonlinear scaling techniques have been shown to be preferable on both theoretical and statistical grounds (Nevill et al., 1992; Welsman et al., in press). Allometric scaling techniques are widely used by comparative physiologists interested in the clarification of structure/function relationships (Schmidt-Nielsen, 1984) and have widespread applications for the interpretation of paediatric exercise data; particularly during growth. One of the key aims of allometric scaling is the identification of the mass exponent which represents size-related function in the population under investigation. Several studies have sought the mass exponent which best describes the relationship between peak $\dot{V}O_2$ and body mass in growing children in order to facilitate the accurate interpretation of the growth of peak aerobic fitness. If peak $\dot{V}O_2$ increased in direct proportion to body mass the allometric equation y= a x mass$^{1.0}$ would be observed i.e., the ratio standard would appropriately normalise data. However, according to theoretical and geometric principles, peak $\dot{V}O_2$ should increase less than proportionately to body mass with a mass exponent of 0.67 (Åstrand and Rodahl, 1986). Indeed, there is now substantial empirical evidence to confirm that this is the case in adult subjects (Nevill et al., 1992; Nevill, 1994a; Åstrand and Rodahl, 1986).

Other authors have disputed this and argued for a mass exponent of 0.75 based upon observations of the relationship between metabolic rate and body mass in various animal species ranging widely in body size (the classic "mouse to elephant" curve) which identified a mass exponent of 0.75 (Kleiber, 1947). Theoretical concepts based upon elastic similarity rather than geometry have subsequently been proffered to explain these empirical findings (McMahon, 1973) and have received some support (Feldman and McMahon, 1983). Others have dismissed the 0.75 exponent as artifactual (Heusner, 1982), criticised the species selection from which it was derived (Calder, 1987) and observed that there is no biologically satisfactory theoretical explanation for it (Heusner, 1987).

To date, the majority of studies reporting the allometric relationship between peak aerobic performance and body mass in children and adolescents have yielded mass exponents which have invariably exceeded 0.67 ranging from 0.88 to 1.07 (McMiken, 1976, Cooper et al., 1984, Paterson et al., 1990, Ross et al., 1991) thus supporting the continued use of the simple ratio standard to normalise peak $\dot{V}O_2$ data in children (Bar-Or, 1983, Shephard, 1982).

Recently a plausible explanation for these elevated exponents has emerged from studies which have demonstrated the pitfalls of generating mass exponents in heterogeneous groups of subjects, specifically groups ranging widely in age and, therefore, size during growth. Alexander (1981) demonstrated that in mammals, proximal leg muscle mass increases disproportionately with the increase in body size: mass$^{1.1}$. A similar relationship has been confirmed in adolescent males with a mass exponent of 1.1 reported for leg volume (Nevill, 1994b). This disproportionate increase in muscle mass with increasing size may be controlled for by incorporating height into the allometric equation when modelling performance measures such as peak $\dot{V}O_2$. By doing so, the independent contribution from body mass may be separated from the confounding influence of the disproportionate increase in muscle mass with increasing body size. These principles have been demonstrated in adult subjects (Nevill, 1994a) and subsequently supported in our study of prepubertal, pubertal and adult males and females (Welsman et al., in press). In this latter study, allometric scaling of peak $\dot{V}O_2$ data revealed a mass exponent of 0.80 common to all groups. However, with height included as a covariate in analysis of covariance on a bilogarithmic plot the mass exponent was reduced to 0.71, a value not significantly different from 0.67. Recently we have presented data which provide fufther empirical support for the argument in favour of a mass exponent of 0.67 to normalise peak $\dot{V}O_2$ data in growing children. In a study of a homogeneous population of 164 prepubertal boys and girls, allometric scaling revealed a common mass exponent of 0.66, almost exactly the value of 0.67 derived from theoretical principles (Welsman and Armstrong, 1995).

The discussion so far has focused upon the appropriate scaling of functional changes in peak aerobic fitness during the period of growth and maturation and provided compelling evidence to support the use of ml x $kg^{-.67}$ x min^{-1} to normalise peak $\dot{V}O_2$ data. This is not to suggest, however, that one particular scaling technique or mass exponent will correctly and adequately partition out body size differences in all analyses of performance. For example, in adults, a ratio standard (ml x kg^{-1} x min^{-1}) best described 5000 m running and sprint performance in adult subjects (Nevill et al. 1992). It should be emphasised that this conclusion was derived from appropriate statistical modelling of the data in question and demonstrates how suitable scaling factors can only be derived from the careful modelling of individual data sets.

In conclusion this discussion has demonstrated the applicability of allometric scaling techniques to the interpretation of peak aerobic fitness in children and adolescents, provided an explanation for the inflated mass exponents previously observed in these age groups and provided strong empirical support for the theoretically derived mass exponent of 0.67 when interpreting peak $\dot{V}O_2$ data. Further research is now required to confirm these suggestions in longitudinal data sets and extend the use of allometric modelling to other performance measures in growing children.

References

Alexander, R. McN., Jayes, A.S. Maloiy, G.M.O. and Wathuta, E.M. (1981). Allometry of the leg muscles of mammals. Journal of the Zoological Society of London, 194: 539-552.

Armstrong, N., Kirby, B., McManus, A. and Welsman, J. Aerobic fitness of pre-pubescent children. Annals of Human Biology, (in press).

Armstrong, N., and Welsman, J. (1994). Assessment and interpretation of aerobic fitness in children and adolescents. Exercise and Sport Sciences Reviews, 22: 435-476.

Armstrong, N., Welsman, J. and Winsley, R. Is peak $\dot{V}O_2$ a maximal index of children's aerobic fitness? (under review).

Armstrong, N., Williams, J., Balding, J., Gentle, P. and Kirby, B. (1991). The peak oxygen uptake of British children with reference to age, sex and sexual maturity. European Journal of Applied Physiology. 62: 369-375.

Åstrand, P.O. (1952). Experimental Studies of Physical Working Capacity in Relation to Sex and Age. Copenhagen, Munksgaard.

Åstrand, P.O. and Rodahl., K. (1986). Textbook of Work Physiology. New York, McGrawHill.

Bar-Or, O. (1983). Pediatric Sports Medicine for the Practitioner, New York: Springer Verlag.

Calder, W.A. III. (1987). Scaling energetics of homeothermic vertebrates: An operational allometry. Annual Review of Physiology 49: 107-120.

Cooper, D.M. and Berman, N. (1995). Ratios and regressions in body size and function: a commentary. Journal of Applied Physiology, 77: 2015-2017.

Cooper, D.M., Weiler-Ravell, D., Whipp, B.J. and Wasserman, K. (1984). Aerobic parameters of exercise as a function of body size during growth in children. Journal of Applied Physiology, 56: 628-634.

Cumming, G.R., Hastman, L., McCoft, J. and McCullough, S. (1980). High serum lactates do occur in children after maximal work. International Journal of Sports Medicine. 1: 66-69.

Cunningham, D.A., MacFarlane, B., Waterschoot, V., Paterson, D.H., Lefcoe, M. and Sangal, S.P. (1977). Reliability and reproducibility of maximal oxygen uptake measurement in children. Medicine and Science in Sports and Exercise, 9: 104-108.

Eston, R.G., Robson, S. and Winter, E.M. (1993). A comparison of oxygen uptake during running in children and adults. In J.W. Duquet and J.A.P. Day (eds.), Kinanthropometry IV, London: E & F Spon, pp. 236-241.

Feldman, H.A. and McMahon, T.A. (1983). The 3/4 mass exponent for energy metabolism is not a statistical artifact. Respiratory Physiology, 52: 149-163.

Freedson, P.S., and Goodman, T.L. (1993). Measurement of oxygen consumption. In T.W. Rowland (ed.). Pediatric Laboratory Exercise Testing. Champaign, Il: Human Kinetics. pp 91-113.

Heusner, A. A. (1982). Energy metabolism and body size, I. Is the 0.75 mass exponent of Kleiber's equation a statistical artifact?: Respiratory Physiology, 48: 1-12.

Heusner, A.A. (1987). What does the power function reveal about structure and function in animals of different size? Annual Reviews in Physiology, 49: 121-133.

Kleiber, M. (1947). Body size and metabolic rate. Physiological Review, 27: 511-541.

Krahenbuhl, G.S., Skinner, J.S. and Kohft, W.M. (1985). Developmental aspects of maximal aerobic power in children. Exercise and Sports Science Reviews, 13: 503-538.

McMahon, T.A. 1973). Size and shape in biology. Elastic criteria impose limits on biological proportions, and consequently on metabolic rates. Science, 174: 1201-1204.

McMiken, D.F. (1976). Maximum aerobic power and physical dimensions of children. Annals of Human Biology, 3: 141-147.

Myers, J., Walsh, D., Buchanan, N., and Froelicher, V.F. (1989). Can maximal cardiopulmonary capacity be recognised by a plateau in oxygen uptake? Chest, 96: 1312-1316.

Myers, J., Walsh, D., Sullivan, M. and Froelicher, V. (1990). Effect of sampling on variability and plateau in oxygen uptake. Journal of Applied Physioliology. 68: 404-410.

Nevill, A. (1994a). The need to scale for differences in body size and mass: An explanation of Kleiber's 0.75 mass exponent. Journal of Applied Physiology, 77: 2870-2873.

Nevill, A. M. (1994b). Evidence of an increasing proportion of leg muscle mass to body mass in male adolescents and its implication on performance. Journal of Sports Science, 12: 163-164.

Nevill, A., Ramsbottom, R. and Williams, C. (1992). Scaling physiological measurements for individuals of different body size. European Journal of Applied Physiology, 65: 110-117.

Noakes,T.D.(1988). Implications of exercise testing for prediction of athletic performance: A contemporary perspective. Medicine and Science in Sports and Exercise,20: 319-330.

Paterson, D.H., McLellan, T.M. Stella, R.S. and Cunningham, D.A. (1987). Longitudinal study of ventilation threshold and maximal O_2 uptake in athletic boys. Journal of Applied Physiology, 62: 2051-2057.

Rivera-Brown, A.M., Rivera, M.A. and Frontera, W.R. (1992). Applicability of criteria for $\dot{V}O_2$ max in active adolescents. Pediatric Exercise Science, 4: 331-339.

Ross, W.D., Bailey, D.A., Mirwald, R.L., Faulkner, R.A., Rasmussen, R, Kerr, D.A. and Stini, W.A. (1991). Allometric relationship of estimated muscle mass and maximal oxygen uptake in boys studied longitudinally age 8 to 16 years. In R. Frenkl and I. Szmodis. (eds.) Children and Exercise, Pediatric Work Physiology XV, Budapest: National Institute for Health Promotion, pp. 135-142.

Rowland, T.W. (1993). Aerobic exercise testing protocols. T.W. Rowland (ed.). Pediatric Laboratory Exercise Testing. Champaign, Il: Human Kinetics, pp 19-4l.

Rowland, T.W. (1993). Does peak $\dot{V}O_2$ reflect $\dot{V}O_2$ max in children? Evidence from supramaximal testing. Medicine and Science in Sports Exercise, 25: 689-693 .

Rowland, T.W. and Cunningham, L.N. (1992). Oxygen uptake plateau during maximal treadmill exercise in children. Chest. 101: 485-489.

Schmidt-Nielsen, K. (1984). Scaling: Why is Animal Size so Important?, Cambridge: Cambridge University Press.

Shephard, R.J. (1982). Physical Activity and Growth, Chicago: Year Book Medical Publishers.

Sjodin, B. and Svedenhag, J. (1992). Oxygen uptake during running as related to body mass in circumpubertal boys: A longitudinal study. European Journal of Applied Physiology, 65: 1-50

Tanner, J.M. (1949) Fallacy of per-weight and per-surface area standards and their relation to spurious correlation. Journal of Applied Physiology, 2: 1-15.

Thoden, J.S. (1991). Testing aerobic power. J.D. MacDougall, H.A. Wenger and H.J. Green (eds.). Physiological Testing of the High Performance Athlete. Champaign, I1: Human Kinetics, pp 107-173.

Toth, M.J., Goran, M.I., Ades, P.A., Howard, D.B. and Poehlman, E.T. (1993). Examination of data normalization procedueres for expressing peak $\dot{V}O_2$ data. Journal of Applied Physiology, 75: 2288-2292.

Welsman, J. and Armstrong, N. (1995). The interpretation of peak volume oxygen ($\dot{V}O_2$) in prepubertal children. In F.J. Ring (Ed.) Children in Sport, Bath: Centre for Continuing Education, pp. 64-69.

Welsman, J. and Armstrong, N. (in press). Post-exercise lactates in children and adolescents. E. van Praagh (ed.), Anaerobic Power and Capacity During Childhood and Adolescence. Champaign, Il., Human Kinetics.

Welsman, J., Armstrong, N. and Kirby, B. (1994). Serum testosterone is not related to peak $\dot{V}O_2$ and submaximal blood lactate responses in 12-16 year old males. Pediatric Exercise Science, 6: 120-127.

Williams, J. and Armstrong, N. (1991). The influence of age and sexual maturation on children's blood lactate responses to exercise. Pediatric Exercise Science, 3: 111-120.

Williams, J., Armstrong, N., Crichton, N. and Winter, E. (1991). Changes in peak oxygen uptake with age and sexual maturation in boys: Physiological fact or statistical anomaly. In J. Coudert and E. van Praagh (eds.), Children and Exercise XVI, Paris: Masson, pp. 35-37.

Winter, E. (1992). Partitioning out differences in size. Pediatric Exercise Science, 4: 296-301.

Winter, E.M., Brookes, F.B.C. and Hamley, E.J. (1991). Maximal exercise performance and lean leg volume in men and women. Journal of Sports Science, 9: 3-13.

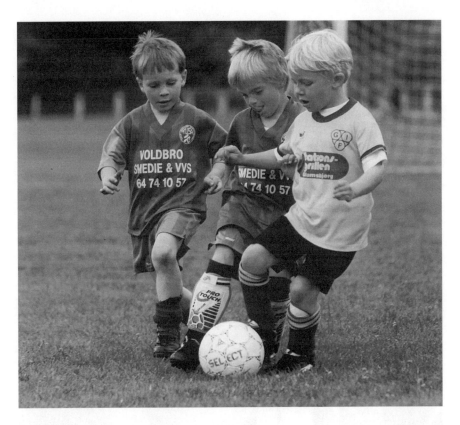

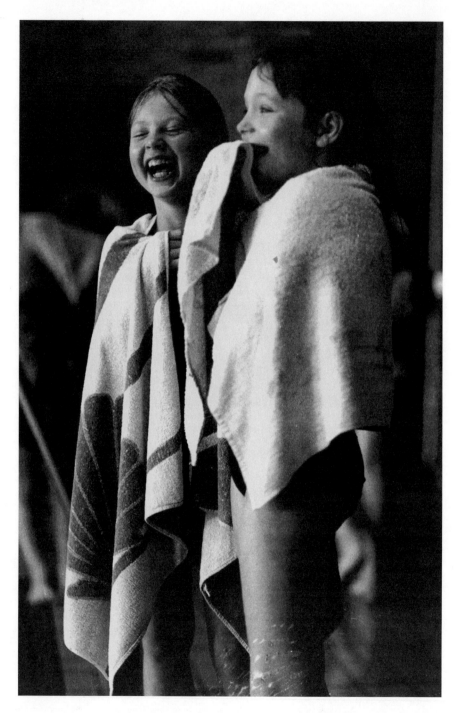

Chapter 13

The Aerobic Trainability of Athletic and Non-athletic Children

Thomas W. Rowland

Changes in the physiologic responses to exercise as children grow – and those separating children from adults – are often related to differences in size alone. That is, maximal oxygen uptake is expected to increase through the course of childhood because the organs responsible for oxygen uptake (heart, lungs, blood volume, skeletal muscle) grow dramatically during this time span. There are, however, certain physiological characteristics of children that appear to be independent of size and are instead more related to level of biological maturation.

The apparent inability of children to improve maximal aerobic power (VO_2max) with endurance training to the extent expected in adults is an example of such a size-independent phenomenon. This discussion will focus on the research data supporting this concept, with extension of the question to include the response to aerobic training by prepubertal endurance athletes. In regards to the latter, the following questions will be addressed:

1. How aerobically "trainable" are prepubertal athletes (i.e., can they improve VO_2max)?
2. Are there quantitative and qualitative differences in response to aerobic training between pre- and post-pubertal athletes?
3. How do such responses in VO_2max translate into changes in endurance performance?

The answers to these questions bear importance to young athletes. Prepubertal athletes are participating at highly competitive levels with training regimens which once would have been considered extreme even for adults. Considerable concern has been voiced regarding the physiological, social, and psychological risks engendered by such training in immature elite athletes. For this reason, recommendations have been made that children avoid intensive specialized training at early ages. If it could be demonstrated that training regimens are not effective in improving aerobic fitness during childhood such recommendations would be supported.

Training in non-athletic children

If a previously sedentary adult is placed in a program of regular endurance training of sufficient intensity, duration, and frequency, a predictable set of cardiovascular changes are observed. These adaptations, termed the "fitness effect", include an increase in maximal stroke volume and cardiac output and decrease in submaximal heart rate. These alterations are manifest as an increase in VO₂max, typically by about 20% in the young adult. Such changes in maximal aerobic power appear to be mirrored by improvements in endurance performance, although the connection between increases in physiologic and performance fitness is poorly understood.

There is no reason a priori to expect that aerobic trainability should be less in children than adults, but evidence suggests this is the case. Bar-Or compiled data on 9 early studies involving children which demonstrated little or no increase in VO₂max (1). It was recognized, though, that many of the studies in this report did not fulfill criteria for type of exercise and duration that would be expected to be necessary (at least in adults) for increasing aerobic fitness with training.

Several authors have more recently assessed the results of those training studies in children, with attention to those which were considered to satisfy such criteria (sustained exercise, three times a week for at least 10 weeks, at prescribed intensity) (11,13,14,19,21,24). Rowland identified 8 such studies, of which 6 demonstrated a significant improvement in VO₂max with endurance training (14). The average improvement in maximal aerobic power was 14 percent. It was concluded that "these data would appear to indicate that when endurance training programs are of sufficient duration and intensity, an improvement in aerobic power in children can be elicited similar to that observed in adults." It was pointed out, however, that these studies suffered from serious methodological weaknesses, including small numbers of subjects, absence of controls, and no documentation of intensity.

Pate and Ward performed a similar review of 12 aerobic training studies in prepubertal children and found an average 10 percent increase (11). Payne and Morrow performed a meta-analysis of 23 pediatric training studies and described an overall rise of only 5 percent (13). Rowland and Boyajian recently described a 6.5% rise in VO₂max in a training study of children specifically designed to avoid the methodological pitfalls of previous investigations (15).

From these data one can reasonably conclude that maximal aerobic power can be improved with endurance training in prepubertal training. However, the magnitude of this response appears to be blunted compared to that expected in adults. If this is true, why should children be different? The influences of training intensity, pre-training levels of VO₂max, and biological factors relative to maturation have all been suggested.

Sufficient exercise intensity is one of the most critical elements of an aerobic training program. There is evidence to suggest that the training intensity, as indicated by heart rate, may need to be higher in children to produce a cardiovascular training effect. This idea comes from data which indicate that the ventilatory anaerobic threshold (VAT) occurs at a higher percentage of VO₂max in children than adults. While controversial, VAT has been considered an appropriate intensity for aerobic training, as it may reflect the optimal level for stressing oxygen delivery. A typical heart rate at VAT for a child is approximately 170 bpm, or 85% of maximal heart rate, considerably greater than that of adults (16). This is a target rate which is higher than that previously utilized in pediatric training studies. It may be that an appropriate comparison of adult and child aerobic trainability can only be performed when training intensity is at a heart rate approximating VAT for each group.

It is well recognized in adults that the magnitude of increase in VO_2max with training is inversely related to the initial maximal aerobic power. That is, the individual with a lower level of aerobic fitness will be expected to show a larger rise in VO_2max with training than the initially more fit subject. Most studies in adults have been conducted in subjects with initial VO_2max levels of 30-45 ml x kg^{-1} x min^{-1}. On the other hand, the children involved in aerobic training studies have typically demonstrated pre-training values of 45-55 ml x kg^{-1} x min^{-1}. Adults who have such high values before training typically only show improvements of about 10%, similar to that seen in children (20). These observations raise the intriguing idea that aerobic responses to training might be similar in children and adults if the two groups were matched for pretraining VO_2max. This possibility is clouded, however, by the question of the appropriateness of using the ratio standard (i.e., expressing VO_2max relative to body mass) to compare aerobic fitness between groups of different sizes (26).

It is possible, too, that biological determinants might be important in reducing the aerobic trainability in children. This is a difficult question to address, since our understanding of the mechanisms which trigger the fitness effect with aerobic training are limited at all ages. We do know that, according to the Fick equation, improvements in VO_2max must reflect increases in maximal heart rate, stroke volume, and/or arteriovenous oxygen difference. Heart rate can be excluded as a possibility, since maximal values do not change significantly with endurance training in either adults or children. Most evidence in adults suggests that maximal cardiac output is the limiting factor in determining VO_2max. It is likely, then, that improvement in maximal stroke volume is the principal factor responsible for changes in maximal aerobic power with training.

There are no reliable data available on stroke volume changes with training in children. Stroke volume can rise from increases in preload (bradycardia, increased plasma volume), improved contractility (by sympathetic or hormonal stimulation), or diminished afterload (fall in peripheral vascular resistance). Decreased submaximal heart rate has been seen in some training studies involving children, but there are no investigations which compare changes in resting heart rate following endurance training with those of adults. Likewise, there is no information available on plasma volume changes with training in prepubertal subjects. Significant increases in plasma volume are observed in adults following a period of aerobic training, which can be manifest in a slight fall in blood hemoglobin concentration. It is of interest, then, that the hemoglobin concentration in child endurance athletes is no different than that of non-athletes. This suggests the possibility that plasma volume changes with training in children could be less than those of adults.

Left ventricular chamber size as measured by echocardiogram has not been shown to be significantly different in children after a period of aerobic training, and resting left ventricular diastolic dimensions of child endurance athletes are not found to be different from non-athletes in most studies (17). This has led to the conclusion that changes in ventricular preload do not contribute to increases in VO2max in children. It should be realized, however, that the changes in stroke volume that would occur with training are of insufficient magnitude to be accurately detected echocardiographically (a 10% increase in stroke volume in a 10-year old child would be manifest by only a 1 mm increase in left ventricular end diastolic diameter if the improvement was due entirely to augmented preload).

Table 1: Biological factors influencing aerobic trainability

1. Increased plasma volume
2. Decreased sympathetic tone
3. Augmented myocardial contractility
4. Diminished ventricular afterload
5. Improved muscle vascularization
6. Increased muscle aerobic capacity

Table 1 lists biological factors which may contribute to the aerobic fitness effect. It is possible to speculate (without any experimental foundation) that a number of these determinants might be affected by maturity-related influences. For instance, children may have a smaller osmotic load with exercise because of lower lactate responses. This could influence factors which stimulate changes in plasma volume. Sympathetic influences with exercise may be less in children. Plasma norepinephrine levels, an index of sympathetic neurological activity, have been reported to be lower in children at maximal exercise in one study (8) but not in another (2). The secretion of testosterone and growth hormone are both dramatically increased at puberty (the former only in males), and these hormones both act to improve myocardial function. How this influence might relate to training, however, is unclear.

In summary, then, VO2max can be improved with endurance training in children, but the magnitude of this response appears to be less than that expected in adults. Intensity of training, differences in pre-training fitness, and biological factors may be responsible for this observation. Puberty may be an important point when aerobic trainability improves. How the limited aerobic response to training in children can be translated into capacity for improvement in endurance performance is unknown.

Aerobic training in child athletes

Against this backdrop of information regarding aerobic trainability in children, it is of interest to examine similar response in child endurance athletes. It is important to recognize at the onset that significant improvements in VO2max are not typically observed in adult endurance athletes who are undergoing training, re-

Table 2: VO₂max studies in male child distance runners.

Study	Age	Mean VO₂max (ml x kg⁻¹ x min⁻¹)
Van Huss et al (25)	9-15	65.9
Daniels & Oldridge (4)	10-15	59.5
Nudel et al (10)	8-17	61.0
Rowland et al (17)	11-13	61.2
Mayers & Gutin	8-11	56.6
Sundberg & Elavainio (23)	12	59.3
Lehamnn et al (8)	12	60.3

flecting the inverse relationship between change in maximal aerobic post and pre-training fitness level. In such adult athletes, however, performance gains are common. While dramatic increases in VO₂max would not, therefore, be expected to be seen in training child athletes, there is evidence that such improvements are, in fact, observed once the age of puberty is reached.

Young endurance athletes clearly have a superior VO₂max when compared to non-athletic children. Table 2 provides data on prepubertal male endurance runners, showing a strikingly similarity of values between studies, typically 60-65 ml x kg⁻¹ x min⁻¹. This represents a 20 percent greater value than that of the average boy, who has a VO₂max of 50-52 ml x kg⁻¹ x min⁻¹. This, of course, does not mean that running training during childhood can improve VO₂max to this extent. It is possible that young athletes simply possess a greater inherent aerobic fitness that has attracted them to sports participation.

There is, however, one observation regarding VO₂max in child endurance athletes that may have some bearing on the trainability question. Note again the remarkable constancy of values for the prepubertal male runners in table 2, supporting the suggestion by Koch that here exists a ceiling of VO₂max from training of about 60 ml x kg⁻¹ x min⁻¹ in young boys (7). Older postpubertal adolescent endurance athletes, on the other hand demonstrate much higher values of VO₂ max, often over 70 ml x kg⁻¹ x min⁻¹ (Table 3). These levels of aerobic fitness are about 60-70% greater than that of the average sedentary adolescent male. This discrepan-

Table 3: VO₂max in male adolescent runners.

Study	Age	VO₂max (ml x kg⁻¹ x min⁻¹)
Kobayashi et al (6)	17	73.9
Dill & Abrams (5)	17	72.0
Cunningham (3)	16	74.6
Sundeberg & Elavainio (23)	16	66.4

cy of VO₂max values between pre- and postpubertal athletes has been interpreted as evidence that children prior to the age of puberty have a dampened capacity for improving VO₂max with endurance training. Alternatively, of course, the older runners may have been trained for a longer period of time, or less fit runners may have dropped out of competition.

From these cross-sectional data, plus what we know regarding aerobic trainability of non-athletic children, it is logical to propose the following hypothesis: Training by endurance athletes prior to the age of puberty does not significantly alter aerobic power. Capacity for increasing VO₂max with athletic training is developed by factors surrounding puberty. To test this hypothesis, three sets of data can be examined, studies testing response of VO₂max in training athletes prior to, after, and through the course of puberty.

Table 4 presents data on three longitudinal studies of VO₂max responses to training in prepubertal athletes. None of these studies included non-training control subjects. Van Huss et al repeated annual determinations of VO₂max for three years in a small number of elite male and female distance runners ages 10-11 and 12-13 years (25). No changes in VO₂max were observed in any of the groups. Similarly, Daniels and Oldridge showed the same stability of VO₂max per kg with distance running in 14 boys ages 10-15 years over 22 months (4). Patterson et al demonstrated an increase in serial testing of prepubertal hockey players, a finding which is difficult to understand considering that hockey training should not be expected to improve aerobic fitness (12).

Table 4: Longitudinal training studies of pre- or early pubertal athletes.

Study	Sport	Controls	Increased VO₂max
Van Huss et al (25)	Distance runners	No	No
Daniels & Oldridge (4)	Distance runners	No	No
Paterson et al (12)	Hockey	Yes	Yes

Two longitudinal studies restricted to postpubertal training endurance athletes both showed significant improvements in massrelative VO2max (table 5). The subjects of Kobayashi et al were 6 highly trained distance runners who had maximal treadmill testing on an annual basis (6). Rusko described improvements in VO₂max in intensely training Finish cyclists and cross country runners (18). The studies of pre- and post-pubertal athletes, then, support the hypothesis.

Two longitudinal studies of athletes training across the pubertal years have provided mixed results. Sjodin and Svedenhag studied 8 young distance runners for 8 years, compared to 4 controls (22). When expressed relative to mass$^{-0.75}$, VO₂max rose significantly over the years in the athletes but not in the controls. The major increase was observed at the age of peak height velocity (indicative of puberty).

Evidence against the hypothesis comes from the report of Zauner et al which describes consistent improvements in VO₂max over three years in young swim-

Table 5: Longitudinal training studies of post-pubertal athletes.

Study	Sport	Controls	Increased VO$_2$max
Kobayashi et al (6)	Distance runners	Yes	Yes
Rusko (18)	Cyclists	No	Yes
	Cros-country skiers		

mers regardless of pubertal status. Testing was performed by treadmill in this study (27).

In summary, then, there is a good deal of supportive-but not conclusive-evidence to support the influence of puberty in promoting aerobic responses to endurance training in athletes. Studies of prepubertal athletes, at least runners, show no appreciable improvements in VO$_2$max with training. How these apparent maturity-related differences in aerobic trainability might be reflected in capacity for improvement in performance is uncertain. As noted previously, failure to increase VO$_2$max with training by adult endurance athletes does not necessarily preclude significant improvements in performance. Whether this is true in prepubertal children remains to be studied.

References

1. Bar-Or, O. Trainability of the prepubescent child. Phys. Sportsmed. 17:65-81, 1989.
2. Charkoudian, N., T.W. Rowland, C.M. Maresh, P.M. Vanderburgh, J.W. Castellani, and L.E. Armstrong. Norepinephrine responses to maximal cycle exercise in boys and men. Med. Sci. Sports Exerc. 27:S94, 1995.
3. Cunningham, L.N. Physiologic comparison of adolescent female and male cross country runners. Pediatr. Exerc. Science 2:313-321, 1990.
4. Daniels, J., and N. Oldridge. Changes in oxygen consumption of young boys during growth and running training. Med. Sci. Sports 3:161-165, 1971.
5. Dill, D.B., and W.C. Adams. Maximal oxygen uptake at sea level and 3,090-m altitude in high school champion runners. J. Appl. Physiol. 30:854-859, 1971.
6. Kobayashi, K., K. Kitamura, M. Miura, H. Sodeyama, Y. Murase, M. Moyashita, and H. Matsui. Aerobic power as related to body growth and training in Japanese boys: a longitudinal study. J. Appl. Physiol. 44:666-672, 1978.
7. Koch, G. Muscle blood flow in prepubertal boys. Effect of growth combined with intensive physical training. In: Medicine and Sport. J. Borms and M. Hebbelink (Eds.) Basel: Karger, 1978, pp. 34-46.
8. Lehmann, M., J. Keul, and U. Korsten-Reck. The influence of graduated treadmill exercise on plasma catecholamines, aerobic and anaerobic capacity in boys and adults. Eur. J. Appl. Physiol. 47:301-311, 1981.
9. Mayers, N., and B. Gutin. Physiological characteristics of elite prepubertal cross country runners. Med. Sci. Sports Exerc. 11:172-176, 1979.
10. Nudel, D.B., I. Hassett, A. Gurain, S. Diamant, E. Weinhouse, and N. Gootman. Young long distance runners: Physiologic characteristics. Clin. Pediatr. 28:500-505, 1989.

11. Pate, R.R., and D.S. Ward. Endurance exercise trainability in children and youth. In: Advances in Sports Medicine and Fitness. Vol. 3. W.A. Grana, J.A. Lombardo, B.J. Sharkey, and J.A. Stone (Eds.) Chicago: Yearbook Medical Publishers, 1990, pp. 37-55.

12. Paterson, D.H., T.M. McLellan, R.S. Stella, and D.A. Cunningham. Longitudinal study of ventilation threshold and maximal O_2 uptake in athletic boys. J. Appl. Physiol. 62:2051-2057, 1987.

13. Payne, V.G., and J.R. Morrow. The effect of physical training on prepubescent VO_2max: a meta-analysis. Res. Q. Exerc. Sport 64:305-313, 1993.

14. Rowland, T.W. Aerobic response to endurance training in prepubescent children: a critical analysis. Med. Sci. Sports Exerc. 17:493-497, 1985.

15. Rowland, T.W. and A. Boyajian. Aerobic response to endurance training in children: magnitude, variability, and gender comparisons. Pediatrics, in press.

16. Rowland, T.W., and G.M. Green. Anaerobic threshold and the determination of target training heart rates in premenarcheal girls. Pediatr. Cardiol. 10:75-79, 1989.

17. Rowland, T.W., V.B. Unnithan, N.G. McFarlane, N.G. Gibson, and J.Y. Paton. Clincal manifestations of the 'athlete's heart, in prepubertal male runners. Int. J. Sports Med. 15:515-519, 1994.

18. Rusko, H.K. Development of aerobic power in relation to age and training in cross-country skiers. Med. Sci. Sports Exerc. 24:1040-1047, 1992.

19. Sady, S. Cardiorespiratory exercise training in children. Clin. Sports Med. 5:493-514, 1986.

20. Saltin, B., L.H. Hartley, A. Kilbom, and I. Astrand. Physical training in sedentary middle-aged and older men. II. Oxygen uptake, heart rate, and blood lactate concentrations at submaximal and maximal exercise. Scand. J. Clin. Lab. Invest. 24:323-334, 1969.

21. Shephard, R.J. Effectiveness of training programmes for prepubescent children. Sports Med. 13:194-213, 1992.

22. Sjodin, B., and J. Svedenhag. Oxygen uptake during running as related to body mass in circumpubertal boys: a longitudinal study. Eur. J. Appl. Physiol. 65:150-157, 1992.

23. Sundberg, S., and R. Elovainio. Cardiorespiratory function in competitive runners aged 12-16 years compared with normal boys. Acta Paediatr. Scand. 71:987-992, 1982.

24. Vaccaro, P., and A. Mahon. Cardiorespiratory responses to endurance training in children. Sports Med. 4:352-363, 1987.

25. Van Huss, W., S.A. Evans, T. Kurowski, D.J. Anderson, R. Allen, and K. Stephens. Physiologic characteristics of male and female age-group runners. In: Competitive Sports for Children and Youth. E.W. Brown and C.F. Branta (Eds.) Champaign, IL: Human Kinetics Publishers, 1988, pp. 143-158.

26. Winter, E. Scaling: Partitioning out differences in size. Pediatr. Exerc. Science 4:296-301, 1992.

27. Zauner, C.W., and N.Y. Benson. Physiological alterations in young swimmers during three years of intensive training. J. Sports Med. 21:179-185, 1981.

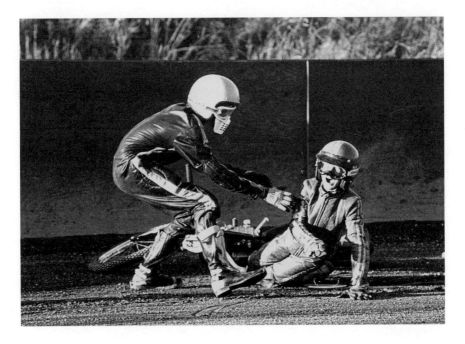

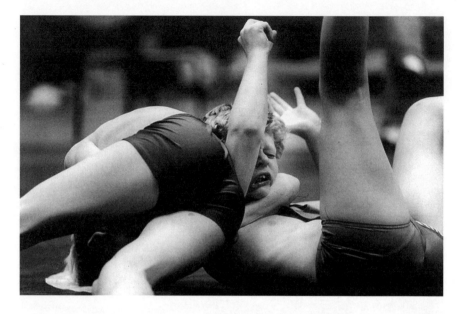

Chapter 14

Muscular Strength Development in Children and Adolescents

Gaston Beunen

Strength as a motor ability usually refers to static or isometric strength in which force is exerted against an external resistance without any change in muscle length. However various indicators of strength have been used (see e.g. Schmidtbleicher, 1984). In the context of epidemiologic studies of growth and development quite often the following strength components are considered: static strength, explosive strength, or power, and dynamic or functional strength. Explosive strength, is the ability of muscles to release maximal force in the shortest possible time. Outside the laboratory, jumping tasks are often used as indicators of this ability. Dynamic strength, sometimes also called functional strength, is the force generated by repetitive contractions of muscles; it is closely linked to muscular endurance which is the ability to maintain or repeat muscular contractions over time. Tests of dynamic, functional strength or muscular endurance include push-ups, pull-ups, sit-ups, curl-ups and flexed arm hang. Factor analytic studies of motor abilities and strength characteristics of boys and girls in the age range 12 to 18 years demonstrate that static strength, explosive strength, functional strength of the upper body and functional strength of the abdominals are fairly independent components of the motor ability domain (Simons et al., 1969, 1978).

The present chapter considers the development from childhood through adolescence of the four "strength" components. Age changes, sexual differences, variation within European populations and changes over time are discussed. Since strength, anthropometric dimensions and biological maturity are interrelated these associations and changes, these associations during the growth process are also described. The chapter builds on earlier reviews and is limited to large epidemiologic fitness studies.

Development of strength and sex differences

In boys, static strength increases fairly linearly with chronological age from early childhood to approximately 12 or 13 years of age, when there is a marked acceleration through the late teens. In girls, strength improves linearly with age through about 15 years, with no clear evidence of an adolescent spurt (Beunen et al. 1988, 1990; Malina and Bouchard, 1991), although some evidence suggest a peak in arm pull strength (Kemper and Verschuur, 1985). This developmental pattern in both sexes is nicely illustrated in a recent study of fitness characteristics of Flemish youth (figure 1a,b). At each age level rather large inter-individual variation is present, but the percentile distribution at each age level is almost symmetric. Evidence from longitudinal studies (Beunen and Malina, 1988) suggests that the adolescent spurt in arm strength begins 1.5 years before age at peak height velocity and reaches a peak about 0.5 years after peak height velocity. The maximum velocity is virtually identical in Dutch and Belgian boys. The estimated velocity of strength development in Belgian Boys is about 30% of attained peak strength, which indicates the marked increase in static strength that occurs in male adolescence. Further, none of the 219 boys followed longitudinally during adolescence have a negative velocity at this time. Similar spurts are found for upper body strength (the average of shoulder extension, wrist flexion and extension, elbow flexion and extension) and lower body strength (average of hip flexion and knee extension) in a sample of 99 Canadian boys. The age at peak strength development is reached 1.0 year after peak height velocity. When strength increments are expressed as a percentage of the level of strength attained, the relative increase is greater for upper body strength than for lower body strength (Carron and Bailey, 1974). In contrast to what has been observed by Faust (1977) in Oakland girls, the timing of the peak arm strength in Dutch girls occurs also 0.5 years after peak height velocity (Kemper and Verschuur, 1985). Peak strength development in Dutch girls is about one-half of that in boys.

On the average, performance in standing long jump and vertical jump increases linearly with age in both sexes until 12 years in girls and until 13 years in boys (Beunen et al., 1988,1990; Malina and Bouchard, 1991). Also, for explosive strength, large inter-individual differences are found as can be seen from the percentile distributions for both sexes of the standing long jump (Figure 1c,d). Again the percentile distributions are symmetric around the median at each age level. For explosive strength a clear adolescent spurt has been demonstrated in Canadian (Ellis, Carron and Bailey, 1975) and Belgian boys (Beunen et al. 1988). Maximum velocity in standing long jump (15 cm x year^{-1} in 106 Canadian boys) coincides with peak height velocity, whereas the maximum velocity in vertical jump (5cm x year^{-1} for 222 Belgian boys) coincides with the maximum velocity in static strength 0.5 years after peak height velocity. The difference in the timing between the Belgian and Canadian study probably reflects analytical differences. In the Belgian study increments were calculated at semi-annual intervals whereas annual increments were used in the Canadian sample.

Changes in functional strength (muscular endurance) as measured by the flexed arm hang are shown in figure 2a,b (page 196). The score for the test is the duration, or length of time that the flexed arm position can be helt until the child's eyes drop below the level of the bar. In boys, the scores change curvilinearly with a marked increase after 12 years, similar to the spurt in static strength. In girls the median scores fluctuate between 4-8 seconds, with no evidence of an adolescent spurt. The percentile distributions in both sexes are markedly skewed and show considerable inter-individual variation. In boys for example the 10% best performers at 6 years obtain a score of about 20 seconds which is about the same score as the median for

Figure 1: Percentile distribution of Flemish boys and girls 6.0 to 18 years by handgrip a. boys, b. girls and standing long jump c. boys, d. girls (after Lefevre et al. 1993, 300 subjects per age category)

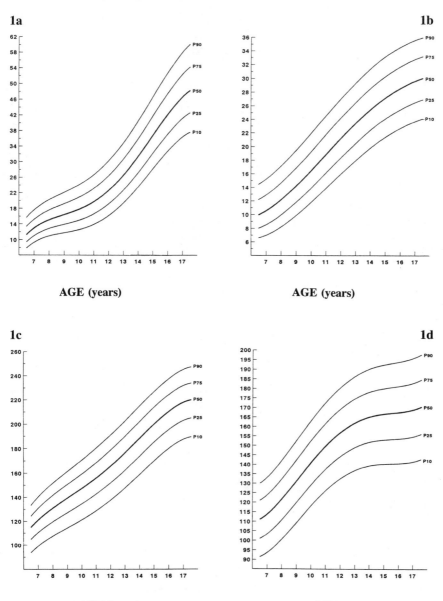

Figure 2: Percentile distribution of Flemish boys and girls 6.0 to 18 years by flexed arm hang a. boys, b. girls and sit ups c. boys, d. girls (after Lefevre et al. 1993, 300 subjects per age category)

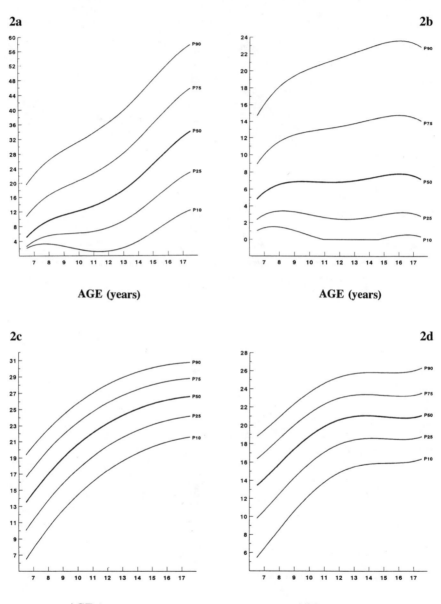

14-year-old boys. Maximum increments (about 5 sec x year⁻¹ in 217 Belgian boys) in flexed arm hang follow peak height velocity and coincide with maximum velocities in static strength (Beunen et al., 1988).

The number of sit-ups increases with advancing age, but in boys the increase gradually declines, whereas in girls there is a slight decrease after 13 years. Contrary to flexed arm hang, percentile distributions are not markedly skewed. Leg lift scores do not show a clear adolescent spurt in Belgian boys followed longitudinally during adolescence (Beunen et al., 1988).

Sex differences in static strength are consistent, though small, through childhood (Malina and Bouchard, 1991). At 13 years the median arm pull scores of girls fall slightly below the median scores of their male peers (figure 3). Thereafter, the differences gradually increase so that at 17 years the median scores of the girls are situated below the 3rd percentile of the boys (Beunen et al., 1989). Similar sex differences are observed for explosive strength, vertical jump and standing long jump, (Beunen et al., 1989; Malina and Bouchard, 1991). In vertical jump, the median score of 13-year-old girls is about the same as the 25th percentile of boys and the differences increase so that at 17 years the girl's median falls below the 3rd percentile of the boys. Sex differences in flexed arm hang are especially apparent after age 8 and gradually increase with increasing age. At 17 years, the median of the girls is situated between the 3rd and 10th percentile of the boys (Beunen et al., 1989). For leg lifts the sex differences are less apparent and the medians at 13 through 17 years for both sexes are nearly identical. For sit-ups, however, similar differences are seen as for the other strength components. These sex differences

Figure 3: Sexual differences in strength components for Belgian youth (after Beunen et al. 1989).

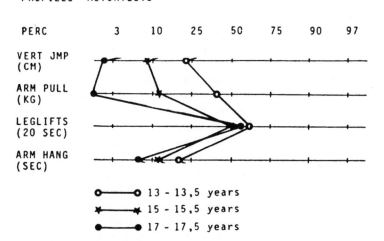

PROFILES MOTORTESTS

Median motor characteristics of 13⁺-, 15⁺-, 17⁺-year-old girls situated within the percentile charts of boys of the respective age levels.

can be mainly explained by the larger muscle mass of boys (Astrand, 1985), although other factors such as differences in daily physical activity, sports practise, and sex roles during female adolescence cannot be ruled out.

Variation in European populations and changes over time

In a recent review of fitness studies of European populations, Beunen et al. (in press) concluded that the growth patterns of the four strength components are strikingly similar across European countries. Strength levels, however differ considerably. The average handgrip scores for all samples of European boys falls well within the means +1SD of Flemish boys. Boys from Hungary and The Netherlands score the highest, while those from Spain and Northern Ireland score lowest (figure 4a). Also, for sit-ups, the results of boys from Northern Ireland, The Netherlands, Iceland, Italy, Spain and Germany fall within the means +1SD of Flemish boys. Italian and Spanish boys score lowest, while boys from Flanders, Germany and Northern Ireland obtain similar results (figure 4b). Flexed arm hang of Flemish, Scottish and Spanish girls are quite similar, while girls from Iceland and to a lesser extent also The Netherlands, obtain better results (figure 4c page 200). For explosive strength (standing long jump), performance scores are variable. The average performances of girls from Iceland differ by more than two standard deviations from the average scores of girls from Northern Ireland, Italy, and Scotland. The results of girls from The Netherlands, Spain and Hungary are situated between those of Flanders and Northern Ireland, Italy and Scotland (figure 4d page 200).

A positive secular trend, i.e. increases over generations in size and maturation, characterize the majority of auxological literature. Positive secular trends in size and biological maturation or the cessation of the trend is found in most developed countries, while data from developing countries illustrate all three types of secular trends. Some segments of the population also show positive secular trends in size and maturity characteristics, while other segments show no secular trend or even a negative secular trend (Malina 1990). Since strength components are part related to size and maturity status, secular increases in size and maturity have implications for strength performance. The relationships between strength characteristics and size and maturity will be discussed in the next section. Malina (1980) demonstrated a marked increase in grip strength measured in the early 1830s and in 1970s in Belgium and in the 1960s in the USA. When expressed per unit stature, strength scores are slightly greater in boys in the 1960s and 1970s up to a stature of approximately 145-150 cm. At greater heights, strength in Belgian boys in the 1830s is greater per unit stature, which probably reflects differences in timing of the adolescent spurt. In contrast, Belgian and American girls in the 1960s and 1970s have greater strength per unit stature than girls in the 1830s. Secular changes in size and strength of Japanese children show similar results. Relative to their stature, Japanese boys and girls in 1929 jumped (standing long jump) better than children in 1969 (Malina 1980). Based on fitness surveys in Belgium conducted between 1969 and 1992 (Hebbelinck and Borms, 1975, Lefevre et al. 1993, Ostyn et al. 1980, Beunen and Simons

Figure 4: Means for European boys and girls a. handgrip, b. sit ups, c. standing long jump and d. flexed arm hang (Flanders : Lefevre et al. 1993; Germany : Crasselt e.a. 1990; Hungary : Barabas 1990; Iceland : Saemundsen 1987; Italy : Marella et al. 1986; Northern Ireland : Riddoch 1989; Scotland : Watkins e.a. 1983; Spain : Prat 1992; The Netherlands : van Mechelen e.a. 1991).

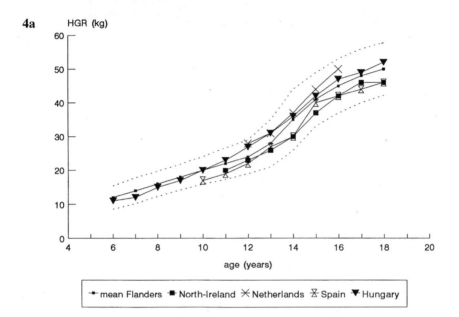

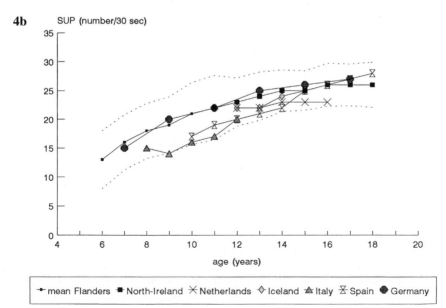

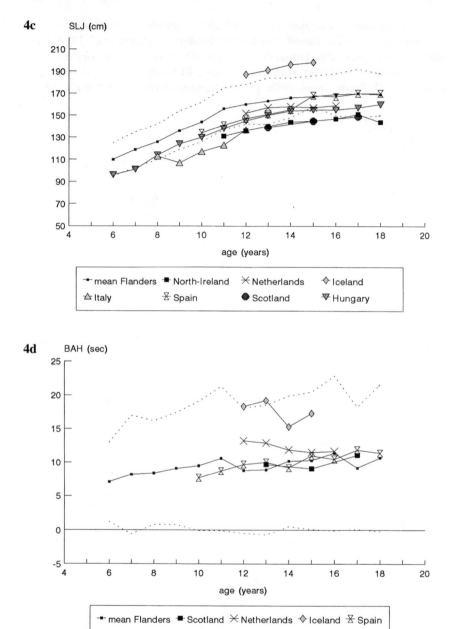

4c   SLJ (cm)

age (years)

| mean Flanders | North-Ireland | Netherlands | Iceland |
| Italy | Spain | Scotland | Hungary |

4d   BAH (sec)

age (years)

| mean Flanders | Scotland | Netherlands | Iceland | Spain |

1990) recent changes in strength characteristics are documented. In boys, handgrip scores did not change between the 1970s and 1990s, while girls scores of the 1970s are greater than those of the 1990s. Considering that in Belgium there is still a slight positive secular trend in stature and weight, relative static strength has decreased in both sexes over the last 20 years. Recent vertical jump scores are identical or slightly higher at older ages than scores observed 10 to 20 years earlier. Sit-ups are also higher in the most recent surveys for both sexes. Also, for flexed arm hang, boys of the 1990s score better than boys of the 1970s. For girls the opposite is found (figure 5a,b,c,d,e,f,g,h pages 201-203). As already mentioned part of the changes over time can be explained by changes in body size and biological maturation. A decrease in physical activity over the last 10 years, especially in late adolescent girls probably has also a negative influence (Taks et al. 1993).

Figure 5. Secular changes in medians for strength characteristics (drawn after data reported by Hebbelinck and Borms 1975; Lefevre et al. 1993; Ostyn et al. 1980; Simons et al. 1990) a. handgrip (HGR) boys, b. handgrip (HGR) girls, c. standing long jump (SBJ) boys, d. standing long jump (SBJ) girls, e. sit upts (SUP) boys, f. sit-ups (SUP) girls, g. flexed arm hang (BAH) boys, h. flexed arm hang (BAH) girls.

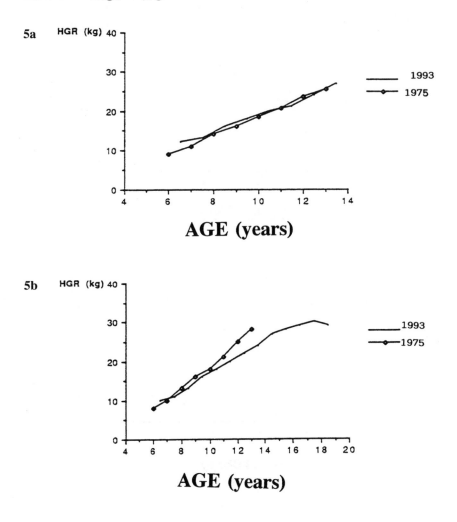

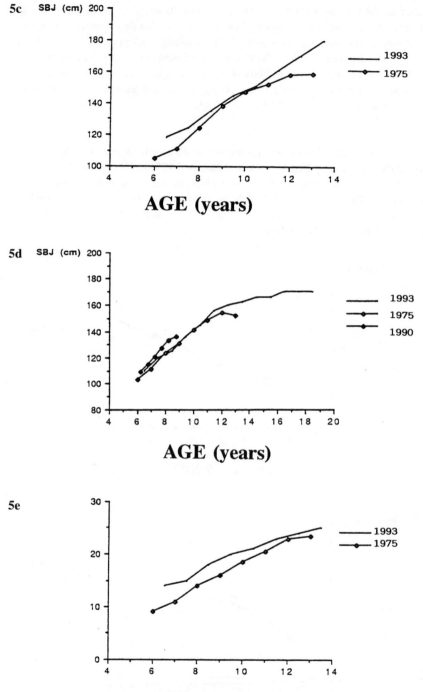

5f

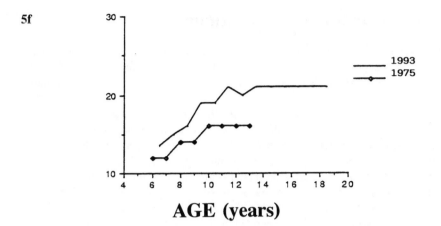

5g

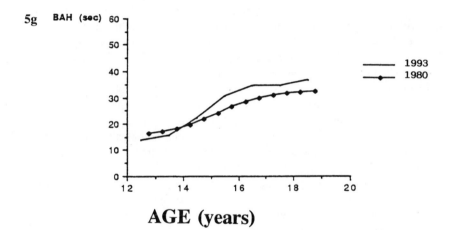

5h

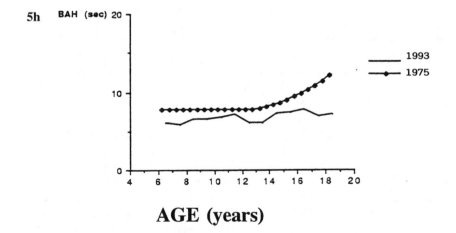

Size and maturity associations

In an extensive review of anthropometric correlates of strength and motor performance Malina (1975) observed that size and maturity are confounded in their effect on performance. It therefore seems of interest to review briefly the available evidence.

Correlations of stature and weight with static strength during childhood fall in the range of 0.30 to 0.60. Thus, the bigger child tends to be the stronger child. The highest correlations occur between 13 and 15 years and reflect individual variation in the timing of the adolescent spurt (Malina and Bouchard, 1991). Correlations for tasks in which the body is projected (standing long jump, vertical jump) or tasks in which the body is raised (push-ups, sit-ups, leg lifts) or supported (flexed arm hang) show consistently negative correlations with body weight, some of which reach into the moderate range (Malina 1994). Physique and static strength are also related during childhood and adolescence. Correlations between static strength and endomorphy and mesomorphy vary between 0.20 and 0.50. Correlations with ectomorphy are negative (Beunen et al. 1985, Malina and Bouchard, 1991). Endomorphy is negatively related with tasks in which the body is projected, raised or supported, while mesomorphy is positively related with such items. Associations with body composition are consistent with those of size and physique. Fatness is positively related to static strength but negatively to the other strength components (Beunen et al., 1983, Malina et al. 1995). When maturity status is controlled, the correlations between strength characteristics, size, physique and composition change. In boys 12 to 18, classified into chronologically and skeletally homogeneous groups, the correlations between static strength and weight vary between 0.44 and 0.54. These correlations are consistently higher than the correlations with stature or other body dimensions, including fatness. Correlations within homogeneous groups for explosive strength, trunk strength and functional strength are lower. Positive, but low correlations are observed between vertical jump scores and body dimensions ranging between 0.0 and 0.22, while correlations with fatness are negative and range between -0.19 and -0.31. Correlations for flexed arm hang and leg lifts on the one hand, and body dimensions and fatness on the other hand are negative and vary between -0.00 and -0.47 (Beunen et al,1984). These results indicate that, when variation in biological maturity is partialled out, correlations change, but the same trends are observed as with the zero-order correlations.

From a recent review concerning the relevance of growth and maturation to athletes (Beunen and Malina, 1995) it can be concluded that, in both sexes, from childhood onwards, static strength is moderately to highly related to indicators of biological maturation. Age-specific correlations vary between 0.35 and 0.81 in boys and between 0.17 and 0.39 in girls. Muscular endurance (functional strength) and trunk strength correlates negatively or non-significantly (age-specific correlations vary between -0.42 and 0.00) in girls, while, in boys, age-specific correlations vary between -0.19 and 0.19. Vertical jump and standing long jump scores are positively associated with biological maturation in both sexes (age-specific correlations vary between 0.00 and 0.48). The correlations are considerably higher when broader age ranges are considered. The association between biological maturation and strength declines considerably when stature and weight are taken into account. This leads to the conclusion that in preadolescents, skeletal age, which is the best single indicator of biological maturity, is not an important predictor of strength. Among adolescent boys, however, correlations between skeletal maturity and static strength and explosive strength are all significant even when chronological age, stature and weight are statistically controlled. Similarly, differences between early and late maturing boys remain significant even when stature and weight are statistically controlled. Finally, there is good evidence that, at least in boys, the strength advantage of early maturers disappears during adulthood (Lefevre et al., 1990). Performances of 30-year-old men grouped on the basis of their age at peak height velocity do not differ significantly for static strength or trunk strength, but late maturers perform better in functional strength (bent arm hang). Late maturing boys improve significantly in strength between 18 and 30 years, more so than early maturing males (Lefevre et al., 1990).

In conclusion, considerable age changes are demonstrated in several strength characteristics with a clear adolescent growth spurt in males for static strength, explosive strength and functional strength. This strength spurt occurs 0.5 to 1.0 year after age at peak height velocity. In girls, an adolescent strength spurt has been observed only for isometric arm strength, although the trend is less clear than in boys. A positive secular trend in strength characteristics has been observed over the last century and also over the last decadest. These changes are reduced or even inversed when secular changes in stature and weight are considered. In both sexes, size, body composition and biological maturation are associated with strength characteristics, although correlations vary with sex, age and strength component.

References

Åstrand, P.O. (1985) Sexual dimorphism in exercise and sport. In J. Ghesquiere, R.D. Martin & F. Newcombe (Eds.) Human Sexual Dimorphism. Symposia of the Society for the Study of Human Biology, 24, London: Taylor & Francis, 247-256.

Barabas, A. (1992) Eurofit and Hungarian school children. In: CDDS, Committee for the Development of Sport. The Eurofit test of physical fitness. VIth European research seminar. Izmir, 26-39 June 1990. Strasbourg: Council of Europe, 223-232.

Beunen, G., Malina, R.M., Ostyn, M., Renson, R., Simons, J. & Van Gerven, D. (1983) Fatness, growth and motor fitness of Belgian Boys 12 through 20 years of age. Human Biology 55, 599-613.

Beunen, G., Ostyn, M., Renson, R.; Simons, J. & Van Gerven, D. (1984) Anthropometric correlates of strength and motor performance in Belgian boys 12 through 18 years of age. In J. Borms, R. Hauspie, A. Sand, C. Suzanne & M. Hebbelinck (Eds) Human Growth and Development, New York: Plenum Press, 503-509.

Beunen, G., Claessens, A., Ostyn, M., Renson, R., Simons, J. & Van Gerven D. (1985) Motor performance as related to somatotype in adolescent boys. In R.A. Binkhorst, H.C.G. Kemper & W.H.M. Saris (Eds.) Children and Exercise XI, Champaign, Ill.: Human Kinetics, 279-284.

Beunen, G., Malina, R.M., Van't Hof, M.A., Simons, J., Ostyn, M., Renson, R. & Van Gerven, D. (1988) Adolescent growth and motor performance. A longitudinal study of Belgian boys. HKP sport science monograph series, Champaign, Ill.: Human Kinetics Books.

Beunen, G. & Malina, R. M. (1988) Growth and physical performance relative to the timing of the adolescent spurt. Exercise and Sport Science Reviews 16, 503-540.

Beunen, G., Colla, R., Simons, J., Claessens, A., Lefevre, J., Renson, R., Van Gerven, D., Vanreusel, B., Wellens, R. & Schueremans, C. (1989) Sexual dimorphism in somatic and motor characteristics. In S. Oseid & K.-H. Carlsen (Eds.) Children and Exercise XIII, Champaign, Human Kinetics, 83-90.

Beunen, G.P. & Simons, J. (1990): Physical growth, maturation and performance. In J. Simons, G.P. Beunen, R. Renson, A.L.M. Claessens, B. Vanreusel & J.A.V. Lefevre (Eds.) Growth and fitness of Flemish girls. The Leuven Growth Study. HKP Sport science monograph series 3, Champaign, ILL: Human Kinetics, 69-118.

Beunen, G. & Malina, R. (1996) Growth and biological maturation: relevance of athletic performance. In O. Bar-Or (Ed.), The Encyclopedia of Sports Medicine: The child and the adolescent athelte, Oxford: Blackwell, 3-24.

Carron, A. V. & Bailey, D. A. (1974) Strength development in boys from 10 through 16 years. Monographs of the Society for Research in Child Development 39 (Serial No. 157).

Crasselt, W., Forchel, I., Kroll, M. & Schulz; A. (1990) (Zum Kinder- und Jugendsport – Realitäten, Wünschen und Tendenzen) Sport for children and adolescents – facts, concerns and trends. Leipzig: Pinkvoss.

Faust, M. S. (1977) Somatic development of adolescent girls. Monograph of the Society for Research in Child Development 42 (Serial No. 169).

Hebbelinck, M. & Borms, J. (1975) (Biometrische studie van een reeks lichaamskenmerken en lichamelijke prestatietests van Belgische kinderen uit het lager onderwijs) Biometric study of a series of body built characteristics and physical performance tests of Belgian children from the primary school. Brussel: Centrum voor Bevolkings- en Gezinsstudiën, Ministerie van Volksgezondheid en van het Gezin.

Kemper, H.C.G. & Verschuur, R. (1985) Motor performance fitness tests. In H.C.G. Kemper (Ed.), Growth, Health and Fitness of Teenagers. Basel: Karger, 96-106.

Lefevre, J., Beunen, G., Steens, G., Claessens, A. & Renson, R. (1990) Motor performance during adolescence and age thirty as related to age at peak height velocity. Annals of Human Biology 17, 434-435.

Lefevre, J., Beunen, G., Borms, J., Vrijens, J, Claessens, A.L. & Van der Aerschot H. (1993) (Eurofit testbatterij. Leidraad bij de testafneming. Referentiewaarden van 6- tot en met 12-jarige jongesn en meisjes in Vlaanderen. Groeicruven voor 6- tot en met 12- jarige jongens en 18-jarige jongens en meisjes in Vlaanderen) Eurofit Testbattery : Guidance for test administration. Reference values for boys and girls 6 to 12 years. Growth curves for Flemish boys and girls 6 to 18 years. Monografie voor Lichamelijke Opvoeding vol. 22. Reeks Sportwetenschappen 2. Gent: Publicatiefonds voor Lichamelijke Opvoeding

Malina, R.M. (1975) Anthropometric correlates of strength and motor performance. Exercise and Sport Sciences Reviews 3, 249-274.

Malina, R.M. (1980) A multidisciplinary, biocultural approach to physical performance. In M. Ostyn, G. Beunen & J. Simons (Eds.) Kinanthropometry II. International series on sport sciences Vol. 9, Baltimore: University Park Press, 33-68.

Malina, R.M. (1990) Research on secular trend in auxology. Anthropologischer Anzeiger 48: 209-227.

Malina, R.M. & C. Bouchard (1991) Growth, Maturation and Physical Activity, Champaign, Ill.: Human Kinetics.

Malina, R.M. (1994) Anthropometry: The individual and the population. Cambridge Studies in Biological Anthropology 14, Cambridge: University Press, 160-177.

Malina, R.M., Beunen, G.P., Claessens, A.L., Lefevre, J., Vanden Eynde, B., Renson, R., Vanreusel, B. & Simons, J. (1995) Fatness and physical fitness in girls 7 to 17 years. Obesity Research 3: 221-231.

Marella, M., Colli, R. & Faina, M. (1986) (Evaluation de l'aptitude physique. Eurofit batterie experimentale) Evaluation of physical fitness. Eurofit experimental battery, Roma: Scuola dello Sport.

Ostyn, M., Simons, J., Beunen, G., Renson, R. & Van Gerven, D. (1980) Somatic and Motor Development of Belgian Secondary Schoolboys. Norms and standards. Leuven: Leuven University press.

Prat, J.A., Casomat, J., Balgue, N., Martinez, M., Povill, J.M., Sanchez, A., Silla, D., Santigosa, S., Perez, G., Riera, J., Vela, J.M. & Portero, P. (1992) (Batterie Eurofit. Standardisation et barèmes basés sur un échantillon de la population Catalane (Espagne)) Eurofit testbattery. Standardization and reference values for a sample of Catalunya (Spain). In: CDDS, Committee for the Development of Sport. The Eurofit test of physical fitness. VIth European research seminar. Izmir, 26-39 June 1990. Strasbourg: Council of Europe, 57-192.

Riddoch, C. (1990) Northern Ireland health and fitness survey – 1989. The fitness, physical activity, attitudes and lifestyles of Northern Ireland post-primary schoolchildren. Belfast: The Queen's University of Belfast.

Saemundsen, G. (1987) Report on the Icelandic experimentation. In: CDDS, Committee for the Development of Sport. 5th European research seminar on testing physical fitness. Scuola Nazionale d'Atletica Leggera, Formia (Italy), 12-17 May 1986. Strasbourg: Council of Europe, 115-127.

Schmidtbleicher, D. (1984) Strukturanalyse der motorischen Eigenschaft Kraft. Lehre der Leichtathletiek. Beilage zur Zeitschrift Leichtathletik 35, 50, 178-179.

Simons, J., Beunen, G., Ostyn, M., Renson, R., Swalus, P., Van Gerven, D. & Willems, E. (1969) (Construction d'un batterie de tests d'aptitude motrice pour garçons de 12 à 19 ans par la méthode de l'analyse factorielle) Construction of a motor fitness test battery for boys of 12 through 19 years of age by factor analyses. Kinanthropologie, 1: 323-362.

Simons, J., Ostyn, M., Beunen, G., Renson, R. & Van Gerven, D. (1978) Factor analytic study of motor ability of Belgian girls, age 12 to 19. In: F. Landry & W.A.R. Orban (Ed.) Biomechanics of sports and kinanthropometry. Miami: Symposia Specialists, 395-401.

Taks, M., Renson, R., Vanreusel, B., Beunen, G., Claessens, A., Colla, M., Lefevre, J., Ostyn, M., Schueremans, C., Simons, J. & Van Gerven, D. (1993) Sociocultural determinants of sport participation among 13 to 18 year old Flemish girls: 1979-1989. In W. Duquet, P. De Knop & L. Bollaert (Eds.) Youth sport. A social approach, Brussel: VUB-Press, 50-58.

van Mechelen, W., van Lier, W.H., Hlobil, H., Crolla, I. & Kemper, H.C.G. (1991) (Eurofit. Handleiding met referentieschalen voor 12- tot en met 16-jarige jongens en meisjes in Nederland) Eurofit. Handbook and reference values for 12- to 16-year-old boys and girls from the Netherlands. Haarlem: De Vrieseborch.

Watkins, J., Farrally, M.R. & Powley, A.E. (1983) The anthropometry and physical fitness of secondary schoolgirls in Strathclyde. Glasgow: Jordanhill College of Education.

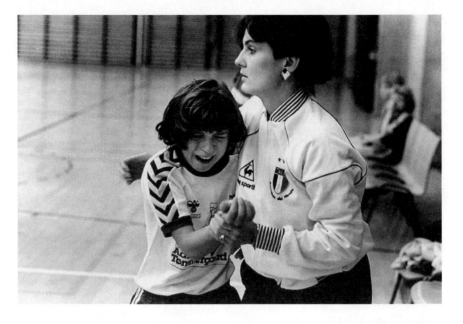

Chapter 15

Etiology and Prevention of Sports Injuries in Youth

Willem van Mechelen

Introduction

During recent decades both the government and sports organizations in the Netherlands have encouraged mass participation in sporting activities, as exemplified by the 'Trim U Fit' (1968), 'Sportreal' (1976), 'Nederland Oké' (1980) and 'Sport, zelfs ik doe het' (1986) campaigns. The Netherlands was not alone in this: witness the 'Sport for All' campaign of the British Sports Council and, again in Britain, the 'Exercise for Health' campaign (Hutson 1983), as well as Fitness Canada (Shephard 1985). Underlying these efforts was the supposedly healthy influence of sporting activities on risk factors, in particular those of cardiovascular diseases.

These efforts have led to an increase in participation in sporting activities in adults.

In children, a shift has been observed from free play in various types of sports and activities to competitive participation in one or two sports.

It is becoming increasingly apparent that these observed changes can present a danger to health in the form of accidents and injuries. A sports person or child who has to give up or cut down his or her sporting activities as a result of an injury is unable to pursue some, or all of his or her goals. If the injury is serious enough, the athlete will have recourse to the medical services to have it treated. Injuries can also result into absence from school or work and even worse to permanent damage.

Given these unwanted side effects of sports participation it was recognized in Europe and elsewhere that a preventive approach towards the reduction of sports injuries should have high priority.

Such measures to prevent sports injuries do not stand by themselves. They form part of what might be called a sequence of prevention (figure 1 page 210).

First, the problem must be identified and described in terms of incidence and severity of sports injuries. Then the factors and mechanisms which play a part in the occurrence of sports injuries have to be identified. The third step is to introduce measures that are likely to reduce the future risk and/or severity of sports injuries. Such measures should be based on the etiologic factors and the mechanisms as identified in the second step. Finally the effect of the measures must be evaluated by repeating the first step.

Figure 1: The sequence of prevention of sports injuries (Van Mechelen et al. 1992)

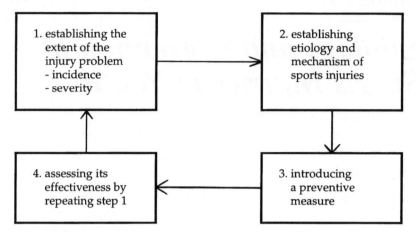

The purpose of this paper is to describe aspects of the etiology and prevention of sports injuries in youth along the lines of the sequence of prevention.

Before doing so, some methodological problems in conjunction with the sequence of prevention will first be discussed.

Methodological problems in sports injury research

The definition of sports injury

In general, sports injury is a collective name for all types of damage that can occur in relation to sporting activities. Various studies of incidence define the term sports injury in different ways. In some studies a sports injury is defined as one sustained during sporting activities for which an insurance claim is submitted; in other studies the definition is confined to injuries treated at a hospital casualty or other medical department (Van Mechelen et al. 1992). Different definitions partly explain the differing incidences found. The results of various sports injury incidence surveys are therefore not comparable. If sports injuries are recorded through the medical channels, a fairly large percentage of serious, predominantly acute injuries will be observed and less serious and/or overuse injuries will not be recorded. If such a limited definition is used, only part of the total sports injury problem is revealed: this 'tip-of-the-iceberg' phenomenon is commonly described in epidemiological research (Walter et al. 1985). This problem is to a large extend found in sport injury epidemiology in youth were a lot of overuse injuries are thought to be found, as well as 'minor' acute injuries.

To make sports injury surveys comparable and to avoid the 'tip-of-the-iceberg' phenomenon as far as possible, an unambiguous, universally applicable definition of sports injury is the first prerequisite. This definition should be based on a concept of health other than that customary in standard medicine, and should for instance, take incapacitation for sports or school into account. Even if one uniform definition of sports injury is applied, the need remains for uniform agreement on other issues, such as the way in which sports injury incidence is expressed, the ways in which reliable estimates are made of both the number of people engaging in sports and the number of injured sports persons.

Sports injury incidence

One way of indicating the extent of the sports injury problem is to count the absolute number of injuries. A way of indicating the relative extend of the problem is to compare the number of sports injuries with for instance the number of road accidents or accidents at work. However the most appropriate indication of disease in the population or a section of the population is incidence. If one substitutes 'sports injury or sports accident' for 'disease', incidence can be defined as the number of new sports injuries or accidents during a particular period divided by the total number of sports persons at the start of the period (population at risk). Incidence also gives an estimate of risk. If one multiplies the obtained figure by 100, one gets the percentage rate (Sturmans 1984). Expressed in this way, sports injury incidence gives insight into the extent of the sports injury problem.

The incidence rate of sports injuries is usually defined as the number of new sports injuries during a particular period (e.g. 1 year) divided by the total number of sports persons at the start of the period (population at risk). Here again, it should be realized that it is important, when interpreting and comparing the various incidence rates, to know what definition of sports injury was used and how comparable were the samples.

Another problem lies in the way incidence rates are expressed. In most cases, the number of injuries in a particular category of sports persons per season or per year is taken, or the number of injuries per player per match. In both examples no allowance is made for any differences in exposure (the number of hours during which the sports person actually runs the risk of being injured), despite the fact that this factor certainly influences the risk of injury. Incidence figures that take no account of exposure are therefore not a good indication of the true extent of the problem, nor can the incidence rates for various sports be properly compared. It would be better to calculate the incidence of sports injuries in relation to exposure time (hours).

The equation of Chambers (1979) recently adapted by De Loës and Goldie (1988) can be used to calculate injury incidence taking exposure into account:

$$\text{Injury incidence} = \frac{(\text{n of sports injuries/year}) \times 10^4}{(\text{no. of participants}) \times (\text{hours of sports participation/week}) \times (\text{weeks of season/year})}$$

Research design

The extent to which sports injury incidence can be assessed depends on: the definition of sports injury; the way in which incidence is expressed; the method used to count injuries; the method to establish the population at risk; and the representativeness of the sample (Kranenborg 1982).

Injuries can be counted retrospectively or prospectively, using questionnaires or person-to-person interviews. Prospective studies can, by quantifying exposure time, accurately estimate the risk and incidence of injury according to the level and type of exposure of an athlete, while retrospective studies can also identify some risk factors depending on choice of research design, e.g. case-control studies (Walter et al. 1985). Case studies have the draw back that no information on the population at risk is available. Therefore, no conclusion can be drawn from case studies, with respect to sports injury incidence, nor with respect to etiology (Walter et al. 1985).

Depending on the methods used the researcher will be confronted to a greater or lesser extent with phenomena such as recall bias, overestimation of the hours of sport participation (Klesges et al. 1990), incomplete responses, non response, invalid injury description and problems related to the duration and cost of research.

Special attention has to be paid to the method of assessing the population at risk and to the representativeness of the sample. If the population at risk is not clearly identified, it is not possible to calculate reliable incidence data. With regard to the representativeness of the sample, it has to be taken into consideration that the performance of sports and therefore the incidence of sports injuries, is highly determined by selection. Bol et al. (1991) recognized 4 different kinds of selection: (a) self-selection (personal preferences) and/or selection by social environment (parents, friends, school, etc.); (b) selection by sports environment (trainer, coach, etc.); (c) selection by sports organizations (organization of competition by age and gender, the setting of participation standards, etc.) and (d) selection by social, medical and biological factors (socio-economic background, mortality, age, aging, gender, etc.). For examples; within a certain sport, competing at a high level increases sports injury incidence; in contrast to individual sports and team sports more injuries are sustained during matches then during training; in contact sports more injuries are sustained than in non contact sports; during and shortly after the growth spurt, boys sustain more injuries.

The severity of sports injuries

A description of the severity of sports injuries is important in making a decision about whether preventive measures are needed, since the need to prevent serious injuries in a particular sport need not to coincide with a high overall incidence of injuries in that sport. The severity of sports injuries can be described on the basis of 6 criteria (Van Mechelen et al. 1992). These criteria will be briefly described below.

Nature of sports injuries

The nature of sports injuries is described in terms of medical diagnosis: sprain (of joint capsule and ligaments), strain (of muscle or tendon), contusion (bruising), dislocation or subluxation, fracture (of bone), etc. It is the nature of the injury that determines whether assistance (medical or otherwise) is sought. Recording of the nature of sports injuries enables the sports with relatively serious injuries to be identified. The nature of sports injuries can also be described according to the injured part of the body.

Duration and nature of treatment
Data on the duration and nature of treatment can be used to determine the severity of an injury more precisely, especially if it is a question of what medical bodies are involved in the treatment and what therapies used.

Sports time lost
It is important for a sports person to be able to take up his or her sport again as soon as possible after an injury. Sport and exercise play an essential part in people's free time and thus influence their mental well-being. The loss of sporting time is an important psycho-social factor. The length of sporting time lost gives the most precise indication of the consequences of an injury to a sports person.

Working or school time lost
Like the cost of medical treatment, the length of working or school time lost gives an indication of the consequences of sports injuries at a societal level. Data of working or school time lost are used to compare the cost to society of sports injuries with that of other situations involving risks, such as traffic accidents.

Permanent damage
The vast majority of sports injuries heal without permanent disability. Serious injuries such as fractures, ligament, tendon and intra-articular injuries, spinal injuries and eye injuries can leave permanent damage (residual symptoms). Excessive delay between the occurrence of an injury and medical assistance can aggravate the injury. If the residual symptoms are slight, they may cause the individual to modify his or her level of sporting activity. In some cases, however, the sports person may have to choose another sport or give up sport altogether. Serious physical damage can cause permanent disability or death, thus reducing or eliminating the individual's capacity for work or school. When taking precautions, then, priority should be given to measures in sports where such serious injuries are common, even though the particular sport it self is characterized by a low incidence of sports injuries and/or a low absolute number of participants.

Costs of sports injuries
The calculation of the costs of sports injuries essentially involves the expression of the above mentioned 5 categories of seriousness of sports injuries in economic terms. The economic costs can be divided into:

1. Direct costs, i.e. the cost of medical treatment (diagnostic expenses such as X-rays, doctor's fee, cost of medicines, admission costs, etc.);
2. Indirect costs, i.e. expenditure incurred in connection with the loss of productivity due to increased morbidity and mortality levels (loss of working time and expertise due to death or handicap).

A conceptual model for the etiology of sports injuries
Risk indicators for sports injuries can be divided into 2 main categories: internal personal risk indicators and external, environmental risk indicators (Van Mechelen

Figure 2: Risk indicators for sports injuries and determinants of sports behavior (Van Mechelen et al. 1992).

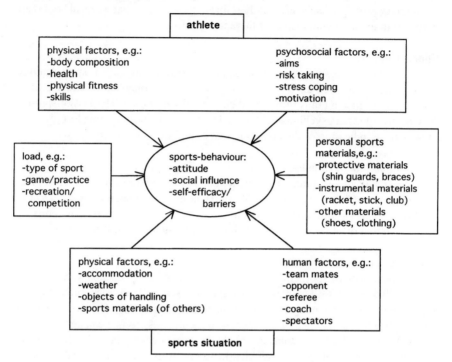

et al. 1992). This division is based on partly proven and partly supposed causal relationships between the risk factors and the injury. However, merely to establish the causes of sports injuries, i.e. the internal and external factors, is not enough; the mechanism by which they occur must also be identified.

Sports injuries result from a complex interaction of identifiable risk factors. Despite this fact most of the epidemiological studies have concentrated on internal and external risk indicators from a medical, monocausal point of view, rather than from a multicausal point of view, that also takes psychological aspects and determinants of sports behavior into account (see figure 2).

To conclude: The outcome of research on the extent of the sports injury problem is highly dependent on the definitions of 'sports injury', 'sports injury incidence' and 'sports participation'. The outcome of sports epidemiology research depends on the research design and methodology, the representativeness of the sample, and whether or not exposure time was considered when calculating incidence. The severity of sports injuries can be expressed by taking six indices into consideration. The etiology of sports injuries is multicausal and should take determinants of sports behavior into account in attempts to solve the sports injury problem.

The etiology and prevention of sports injuries in youth

Children participate in sports in various ways. At a younger age they are pre-domi-nantly engaged in free play activity, school physical education lessons and non or-ganized sports activities. As they grow older they move away from free play and get involved in organized sports activities. Obviously in all these activities children sustain the risk of getting injured. However, there are differences; free play acti-vity, school physical education lessons and non organized sports activities tend to lead to traumatic (acute) sports injuries. Organized sports activities, however, may provide a greater chance to sustain overuse injuries due to the repetitive strain placed upon tissues by the involvement in one or two specific sports and by ad-vancing the duration and intensity of specialized training.

Information on traumatic sports injuries in children comes from epidemiologi-cal studies. The majority of the epidemiological studies give little information about overuse injuries, as a result of the methodology used in these studies. What we know about overuse injuries in youth comes mostly from case studies.

Given this fundamental difference in research design these two types of injuries will be discussed in seperate sections.

Incidence of acute sports injuries in youth

There are no data about the absolute number of acute sports injuries in youth with-in society. Few data are available comparing the extent of the sports injury problem in children to that of other activities of daily life, such as traffic. One of the few studies addressing this issue is that of Guyer and Ellers (1990). They estimated that in 1985, sports contributed third to all hospital inpatient treatment in the US and for about 15% to 16% of all emergency department treatments in children aged 0-19 years, whereas falls, not related to sports, accounted second for 21% and 23% respectively. In the majority of the cases (30% and 49% respectively), the reason for injury was unknown.

Those studies that do calculate the incidence of sports injuries in children show different data due to differences in definitions, design and population. For instance in a population study in the Netherlands (Van Galen and Diederiks 1990), an inju-ry was defined as any self-reported injury sustained in organized and non orga-nized sports, leaving injuries during school physical edication lessons out of con-sideration. In this study, a retrospective study design with a 4 week recall period was applied. For children the following injury incidences per 1000 hours of sports participation were found: 0-4 years 1.8, 5-9 years 1.4, 10-14 years 3.8 and 15-19 years 3.9. After the age of 19, the sports injury incidence rose to 4.3 injuries per 1000 hours of sports participation by the age of 25-29 years, then decreased to 1.9 by the age of 50-54 years. In their study, sex, exposure time, type of sport and in-tensity of play proved to be independent risk factors after multivariate analysis, whereas age was not.

In the Netherlands, amongst 7468 school-aged children (8-17 years) an inci-dence was found of 10.6% in a retrospective survey with a six weeks recall period (Backx et al. 1989). In this study a sports injury was defined as any physical damage caused by a sports-related incident and reported as such. The authors stated that this incidence figure was high for such a short recall period, but attributed this finding to their broad definition of sports injury. They clearly demonstrated a significant age effect (the older one gets the more injuries one sustains), as well as a significant sex effect (girls having a 1.4 greater risk than boys) and a significant effect of the intensity of play (the greater the intensity, the bigger the chance to sustain an injury). However, their data were not corrected for the possible influence of differences in exposure time that may for instance exist between boys and girls, or amongst the various age groups. A second criticism is that they applied univariate statistics on a multicausal health problem, thereby not accounting for the influence of an interaction that may exist between for instance, age and level of activity (perhaps younger children play at a lower level of intensity than older children).

In a second study of Backx et al. (1991a) again incidence and severity of sports injuries was studied. This time it concerned a 7 months prospective study on a sample of 1818 school children aged 8-17 years drawn from their 1989 study. Injury was defined as any damage caused by an accident during physical education lessons or any other sports event outside school. Also exposure time was assessed. They counted 399 injuries in 324 children and found 1 year incidence rates to vary per sport: children playing organized forms of basketball, handball and korfball sustained 1 injury per year. Volleyball, field hockey and soccer had a incidence rate of 50%, whereas physical education lessons showed a incidence rate in 1 out of every 9 children. The overall 7-months injury incidence rate was 22%. Incidence rates expressed per exposure time showed that the rates in games were about three times as high compared to practice. Sports particularly at risk were the contact sports.

The influence of exposure time on the interpretation of injury incidence data was clearly demonstrated by Zarycznyj et al. (1980), who performed a one year prospective study on sports-related injuries in school-aged children in a community of 100,000 inhabitants in the USA. In this study, a sports injury was defined as any traumatic act against the body sufficiently serious to have required first aid, filling of school or insurance reports, or medical treatment. In this population, containing 25,512 children, 1495 sports injuries were registered. Consequently a yearly sports injury incidence rate of 6% was calculated. Since exposure time in this

Table 1: The absolute number of injuries (n), the participant injury incidence rate (%) and the injury incidence (i) per 1000 hours of organized sports participation (i/1000 hours) for five specific sports.

sport	n	%	i/1000 hours
American football	126	28.3	1.05
basketball	29	10.2	0.30
wrestling	27	16.4	0.54
track and field	23	7.9	5.68
baseball	13	9.5	0.52

study was known for all organized sports participation, they were able to present the absolute number of injuries, the participant injury incidence and the injury incidence per 1000 hours of sports participation for specific organized sports (table 1).

In their study Zarycznyj et al. (1980) also showed differences according to age and sex, and according to the level of organization (e.g. school teams, non-organized sports, physical education lessons and community teams), but again, in the absence of information on the extent of the exposure time, it cannot be judged whether these differences are "true" differences.

Tursz and Crost (1986) performed a 1 year prospective study in which they collected data on all accidents involving children aged 0 to 15 years reported to a medical facility in a health care district. The population at risk consisted of about 103,000 subjects. An injury was defined as an unexpected, unintended and violent event affecting the child, with or without detectable lesion, and subsequently leading to medical attention. They counted 7182 accident cases, of which 789 were sports injuries. Although precise information of the population at risk was not available a yearly sports injury incidence rate of 1% was estimated.

Watson (1984) followed 6799 school children, aged 10-18 years, for one academic year. No clear definition of injury was given, but the definition was presumably based on whether or not medical treatment had taken place. Injuries were recorded by the physical education teachers of the school attended by the children. A yearly sports injury incidence of 2.94% was calculated.

In a 2 year prospective study in a group of 453 elite athletes aged 8-16 years, a sports injury was defined as any injury as a result of sports participation with one or more of the following consequences: a reduction in the amount or level of sports activity and a need for medical treatment (Baxter-Jones 1993). In this study, the 1 year incidence was 40 injuries per 100 children. Since training time was known the incidence per 1000 hours training time was calculated. It was found to be less than one injury per 1000 hours of training. There were no sex differences, but there were differences according to type of sport, and most injuries were sustained during training. However, these differences were not corrected for differences in exposure time. In 2 years, 492 injuries were registered of which 148 were classified as overuse. The findings concerning these overuse injuries will be discussed in the section on overuse injuries.

Recently De Loës (1995) reported the results of an analysis of sports injury incidence in a nationwide Swiss youth organization. It concerned medically treated sports injuries for which an insurance claim was made with the sports organization. In three years following 1987 some 5000 injuries were registered annually in about 350,000 boys and girls aged 14-20 years, participating in 32 different sports. The over-all sports injury incidence rate was 4.6 injuries per 10,000 hours of sports participation. Major differences in injury incidence rates were found according to sport; the highest rates were found in contact-sports (ice-hockey 8.6 injuries per 10.000 hours; handball 7.2 injuries per 10,000 hours; soccer 6.6 injuries per 10,000 hours). Significant differences were found between males and females (females having higher incidences in 4 of these sports) when injury incidence rates were calculated for 11 sports in which both males and females participated. However, when the data were standardized for differences in exposure time, and when leaving out soccer, no differences between males and females were found. This is in line with the findings of Macera and Wooten (1994) who also found no gender differences in injury incidence in a review of the literature. De Loës (1995) also clearly showed sports specific differences in incidence rates when incidence was calculated according to medical diagnosis.

Severity of acute sports injuries in youth
As indicated in section 4 the severity of sports injuries can be described using 6 different indices.

The nature of acute sports in terms of medical diagnosis is not consistently reported in the literature. In the study of Zaricznyj et al (1980) 80% of the injuries consisted of sprains, contusions, lacerations and superficial injuries. The remaining 20% were mostly fractures. Findings on the medical diagnosis of sports injuries were also reported by Watson (1984), Tursz and Crost (1986), Backx et al. (1989) and Backx et al. (1991a). All these studies give different frequencies of the above mentioned medical diagnosis (table 2).

Table 2: The nature of acute sports injuries in children according to medical diagnosis (n.a.= not applicable).

Medical diagnosis	Zaricznyi et al 1980	Watson 1984	Tursz and Crost 1986	Backx et al 1989	Backx et al 1991a
contusion		12%	45%	40%	43%
cuts, laceration	80%	9%	16%	n.a.	7%
sprain, strain		41%	17%	44%	30%
fractures	16%	17%	22%	6%*	7%*
other	4%	21%	0%	10%	20%

* incl. dislocations

All these studies also observed, differences in the number of specific injuries per sport, level of participation, intensity of play, age, sex, etc., but in absence of denominator data, it is hard to interpret these differences. Thus it must be questioned whether these differences are true differences, or the consequence of the methodological differences between the studies involved.

Table 3 presents information on the nature of acute sports injuries in children according to the affected part of the body. Here again one is faced with differences between the various studies.

In the study of Zaricznyj et al (1980) 20% (n=312) of all injuries were considered being serious and in need of extensive medical treatment; 4% of all injuries led to hospitalization and 1.2% of all injuries led to permanent damage.

In the study of Watson (1984), the recorded injury (n=116) resulted on the average in 0.47 days of hospitalization, 18 days of incapacity and 29 days before full re-

Table 3: The nature of acute sports injuries in children according to the affected part of the body (n.a.= not applicable).

Medical diagnosis	Zaricznyi et al 1980	Tursz and Crost 1986	Backx et al 1989	Backx et al 1991a
head	20%	14%	5%	6%
trunk	6%	7%	7%	3%
upper extremity	41%	43%	20%	19%
lower extremity	33%	28%	68%	69%
other	n.a.	8%	n.a.	n.a.

covery. In the study from Tursz and Crost (1986) 64% (n=505) of all injuries needed ambulatory medical care. Hospitalization was needed in 11% of all injuries. The average total length of stay in the hospital was 6.9 days and the percentage of stays of 6 days or more was 36%. In 12% of the inpatient cases, residual deformities of the musculo-skeletal system and limitation of articular mobility were observed.

Backx et al. (1989) measured the consequences of sports injuries in children in three ways: subsequent non-attendance of p.e.-classes, non-attendance of school and/or the need for medical treatment. Of all injuries (n=791) 36% led to non-attendance in physical education classes, 6% to non-attendance at school and 31% needed medical treatment. In their 1991 follow-up study, the following was found: non-attendance of physical education classes longer than 1 week 18%, non-attendance in school longer than 1 day 8% and medical treatment 25%.

With the exception of the information given by Guyer and Ellers (1990) little is known about the cost of sports injuries in children. These authors estimated the total cost of hospital inpatient and emergency department treatment of children (0 to 19 years) in the US in 1982 as a result of sports injuries to be US$ 580.8 million of a total of US$ 7544.9 million, ranking third after traffic-related injuries (US$ 2785.2 million) and injuries as a result of a fall (US$ 809.6).

Etiology and prevention of acute sports injuries in youth
Given the multicausal origin of sports injuries epidemiological studies it is vital that studies on the etiology include multivariate statistical techniques. However, with the exception of the study of Backx et al (1991a), none of the other epidemiological studies on the etiology of sports injuries in children applied such analyses. This limitation should be kept in mind when interpreting the information given below.

In the study of Zaricznyj et al (1980) 27% of the injuries were judged as "avoidable", which means that standard safety procedures had not been applied, either from the side of the child, or from the side of the trainer, parent or coach; 40% of those injuries were caused by the child, 30% were caused by improper actions of other players, 20% resulted from a collision with obstacles, and less than 10% of the injuries were caused by improper playing surfaces. Only two injuries were the result of equipment failure. Over 50% of the avoidable injuries occurred during non organized sports and one third during physical education lessons. Only 13% occurred in organized sports. Based on these findings Zaricznyj et al (1980) suggested the following preventive measures; "adequate training", "the use of protective devices", "supervision in injury prevention" and "the transfer of principles and habits of safety learned during physical education lessons to non organized sports activities".

Watson (1984) identified the following major contributory factors on the incidence of sports injuries in children: "recklessness on the part of the injured subject" (26%), "foul or illegal play by another player" (25%), "inadequate sports gear, foot wear, playing areas and equipment" (13%) and "a lack of fitness" (9%). In 63% of all injuries more than one factor was identified as a major cause. As preventive measures, Watson emphasized the limits of safety in individual sports, an active discouragement of recklessness and athletically counter-productive behavior, and a strict application of rules by referees and harder penalties for rule offenders.

Tursz and Crost (1986) found that in 58% of the injuries, a fall was the cause of the injury, in 16% of the cases the child was struck by an object and in 9% by another child. They stated that there was no involvement of other children or sports equipment in most of the cases of injury. Based on these findings, they suggested that preventive measures should focus on children's teaching and training rather than on changes in equipment.

The study of Backx et al. (1989) has listed the causes of 791 sports injuries as follows: misstep/twisting motion (31%), falling/stumbling (24%), kick (13%), ball (11%), opponent (10%), tiredness (3%) and unknown (12%). In some cases, a combination of factors was involved. Based on these findings, Backx et al. (1989) concluded that intrinsic factors, such as joint stability and physical fitness, are much more important than extrinsic factors such as the trainer, the referee, the opponent or sports materials.

In the follow-up study, Backx et al. (1991a) mentioned the following causal factors for sports injuries: falling/stumbling (24%), misstep/twist (22%) and kick/-push (18%). In their analyses of etiologic factors, they found that age, gender and school level were not related to injury. They claimed the nature and extent of sports participation to be of major importance. They found the season to influence the injury pattern, but not the injury incidence calculated according to exposure. In spring, more sprains of the ankle and fractures of the distal parts of the upper limbs were observed. Injuries sustained in spring were more severe in terms of a longer duration of injury. In the multiple regression analysis, the following factors were found to explain 78% of the injury variance: outdoor sports, sports with a high jump rate and sports with physical contact. In their study they found, in terms of the absolute number of injuries, differences in injury pattern between the various sports activities; e.g. more ankle sprains in organized sports and more upper extremity injuries in physical education lessons. The latter also gave rise to more serious injuries than injuries sustained in the other sports categories. They attributed these differences to differences in the quality and extent of the supervision. They also argued that the chance to sustain an injury is predominantly sport related and also depended on the actual exposure time itself. Based on their findings they proposed the following preventive measures: the use of protective equipment, a change in personal sports behavior, a change of rules in order to reduce contact, the inclusion of training, physical education lessons of the teaching of falling techniques and of muscle strengthening and coordination exercises, the latter with an emphasis on ankle training. It was also suggested to incorporate these measures in a theoretical framework provided to the children in cooperation with biology teachers.

In line with these recommendations Backx (1991b) introduced a 4 months preventive programme to a group of 384 schoolchildren (boys and girls) with an average age of 13.6 years, containing the following measures; warming-up, stretching exercises, cooling-down, exercises for stabilization of the ankles, exercises for general coordination and techniques to fall correctly. The measures were provided to the children both in theory during biology lessons and in practice during regular physical education lessons. When evaluating the effectiveness of this controlled intervention study a significant change in both knowledge and attitude with respect to injury prevention was found in this group of school children. However these changes explained only 2% of the variance of the injuries sustained during follow-up.

The above given findings are all derived from studies that, to greater or lesser extent, can be characterized as population or schoolbased studies. Recently some prospective studies have been completed that concern specific etiologic factors studied in specific populations.

Stuart and Smith (1995) found in a 3 year prospective study amongst 17-20 year old ice hockey players a striking difference in injury incidence between training and game; 9.4 injuries per 1000 player practice hours versus 96.1 injuries per 1000 player game hours. They also found defense men to have a smaller injury risk during games than players at other positions. No differences were found during practice. The most common injuries were facial lacerations and acromioclavicular joint injuries. Based on their findings they proposed the following preventive measures: mandatory full facial protection, enforcement of existing rules, improvement of shoulder pad design and the introduction of stretching programs.

Kaplan et al. (1995) followed 2 high school American football teams for 1 season to study the question whether obesity is a risk factor for musculo-skeletal injury or not. In 98 players with an average age of 16.6 years they found an overall incidence rate of 0.29 injuries per player season. They were not able to confirm the independent contribution of obesity to an enhanced injury risk. However, in their study, high body mass as such (>90 kg.) was associated with a 2.5 times higher relative risk of injury. It should be noted that in this study no correction was made for differences in exposure time. This may have influenced the results.

Linder et al. (1995) followed 340 adolescent junior high school American football players aged 11-15 years for 2 seasons. The purpose of their study was to determine the influence of sexual maturity on the risk of sustaining acute sports injuries. It is often debated that with children of the same calendar age, the less mature player has a greater risk of sustaining an injury due to the inequality in body dimensions. They found an overale injury incidence rate of 16%, with an increased injury risk for boys in Tanner stages 3, 4 and 5 (which was in contrast to the expectations). These findings were explained by the fact that more mature boys are perhaps more aggressive because of their advanced growth, and are therefore more susceptible to sustain injuries. Also, the discrepancy in growth rate between bony and soft tissue (see also paragraph 2) may explain this finding. Unfortunately these data were not corrected for differences in exposure time. It may well have been that less mature players were, because of their physique, allowed less playing time than more mature players.

A great number of measures to prevent sports injuries in children have been suggested in a "Current Comment" of the American College of Sports Medicine (Smith et al. 1993). With respect to acute sports injuries, these measures concern the application of a warm-up, the enhancement of compliance with (safety) rules, the improvement of adult knowledge about game rules, equipment and healthy sports behavior and the qualification of coaches and trainers. Also measures like the modification of rules according to the physique of the participants, the avoidance of excessive pressure from parents on winning and to emphasize aspects of play and fun, the counseling of children towards sports that are realistic given the individuals body type and dimensions, the use and maintenance of equipment that meets certain safety rules and the supervision of all competitive sports are advocated. It is clear that these measure are logical and plausible. The 'true' effect of many of these measures has, however, yet to be established.

Overuse sports injuries in youth
General description
According to Micheli and Klein (1991) and Gerrard (1993), overuse injuries in children are due to the repetitive training young children undergo in a single sports discipline. This kind of training leads to repetitive micro-trauma and eventually to overuse injuries when the basal ability of the tissue to repair itself is outplaced by the repetition of insults (Micheli and Fehlandt 1992). These injuries concern predominantly muscle-tendon-bone structures. The ultimate example of such an injury sustained by a child is the case of "Nintendinitis", an overuse injury of the thumb due to playing Nintendo gameboy, reported by Micheli and Fehlandt (1992).

According to Stanitsky (1988), about two-thirds of the overuse injuries in children is related to exertional injuries typically found in older athletes (stress fractures). In the remaining one third, the symptoms are typical of a syndrome proportional to age. This section will further restrict itself to these syndromes proportional to age.

The fact that growing bones are 2-5 times as weak as muscle, ligaments and tendons is an important contributory factor to the etiology of overuse injuries in children (Micheli and Klein 1991, Maffulli 1992, Gerrard 1993, Meyers 1993, Macera and Wooten 1995). In the immature skeleton, growth cartilage is found in the growth plate (physis) of the long bone (figure 3). Growth cartilage is also found at the articular surface (epiphysis) and at the site of attachment of tendons to the bone (apophysis). The physis separates the epiphysis from the metaphysis, the remainder of the long bone (Micheli and Klein 1991, Gerrard 1993).

The physis is less resistant to torsion and shear forces than the surrounding bone and is therefore at risk for injury. The articular surface in children seems vulnerable to fracture due to direct trauma. Repetitive micro trauma of the apophysis leads to tiny avulsion fractures of the apophyseal plate with subsequent inflammatory changes. As a result of the growth process specific injuries are seen in children: growth plate fractures, epiphyseal fractures, osteochondrosis dissecans and traction apophysitis (Maffulli 1992, Micheli and Fehlandt 1992, Meyers 1993, Macera and Wooten 1995).

Epiphyseal plate closure is recognized as the end stage of bony maturation. If an injury to the physis or the epiphysis is sustained before epiphyseal plate closure then a long-term follow-up is required to detect possible growth disturbances (Gerrard 1993, Meyers 1993).

Next to growth, another risk factor for overuse injuries in children is the growth spurt itself. During the growth spurt the bone grows faster than the tendons and ligaments. This leads to decreased flexibility of the muscles, an increase of stress to the site of attachment of ligaments to the bone, and to an increased risk of traction apophysitis (Meyers 1993). The apophysis becomes the weakest link in the tightened muscle-tendon unit, with subsequent injury and inflammation: apophysitis (Micheli and Fehlandt 1992). Growth spurt in boys starts 1 to 2 years later than in girls, who reach puberty earlier. From 12 to 14 years, girls look taller and are often heavier than boys. Beginning their growth spurt later, boys experience a greater acceleration of growth that lasts for several years longer than in girls, whom they surpass in height by the age of 15-16 years, at which time girls

Figure 3: Location of growth cartilage – sites of potential overuse injury (modified from Micheli and Klein 1991, Gerrard 1993).

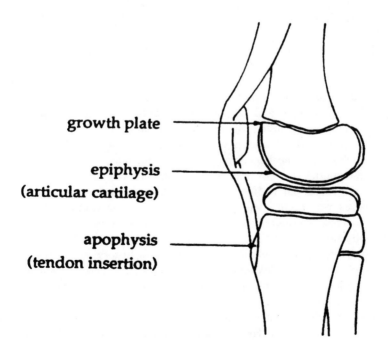

growth plate

epiphysis
(articular cartilage)

apophysis
(tendon insertion)

have reached their adult height. Adult height is reached by boys at the age of 18 years (Micheli and Fehlandt 1992). Meyers (1993) has indicated that the risk of sustaining epiphyseal injuries in boys is greatest in Tanner stages 2 and 3 and in girls in stages 3 and 4, representing the periods of most rapid growth.

Epidemiological data on overuse injuries in children

Almost all of the available information on overuse injuries in children is either based on case studies or common clinical sense, with the exception of the study of Baxter-Jones et al. (1993).

In the prospective study of Baxter-Jones et al. (1993) in elite athletes, one third of the injuries (n=148) was found to be of an overuse nature. Overuse was defined as any injury for which the subject was unable to remember a clear onset. Of 52% of these injuries, the diagnosis could not be specified, the other 48% were specified as follows: osteochondrosis 26%, low back pain 13%, muscle strain 4%, stress fracture 3%, epiphyseal injury 1% and spondylolysis 1%. They found an equal likelihood between the sexes to sustain overuse injuries, but found differences between sports, with swimmers being most at risk. Overuse injuries in this study were more severe than acute injuries: the lay off time for sports participation due to overuse injuries was 20 days compared to 13 days for acute injuries. They also tried to relate pubertal status to the risk of sustaining injuries, but found no relation. Based on their findings they suggested as a preventive measure, a reduction of training intensity, specially during periods of rapid growth.

In the earlier described study of Tursz and Crost (1986) on a total of 789 sports injuries only 10 epiphyseal fractures were observed.

Without indicating his precise source Stanitsky (1989) states that many of the overuse injuries in children are seen in inactive individuals, for whom any athletic stimulus may result in athletic overuse musculo-skeletal complaint.

Micheli and Fehlandt (1992) have described a retrospective analysis of a series of 445 cases of tendinitis and apophysitis in children aged 8-19 years treated in a children's hospital between 1980 and 1990. It should be stressed that data from case series are difficult to interpret given the absence of denominator data (Walter et al. 1985, van Mechelen 1992). Despite this drawback, some information can be obtained from that study. In their sample, Micheli and Fehlandt (1992) found 139 apophyseal injuries and 595 cases of tendinitis. It concerned diagnosis such as tendinitis of the wrist, calcaneal apophysitis, achilles tendinitis, iliac apophysitis, etc. Most of these injuries (n=636) were sustained on the lower extremity. No gender differences were observed. In 50% of the 192 male cases, multiple overuse injuries were diagnosed, whereas this was the case in 38% of the female cases. An example of multiple overuse injuries regularly observed in this case series was the combination of patella tendinitis and tibila tubercle apophysitis. In most of the injuries the authors observed supposed etiological factors as: a history of overuse due to sports, muscle tightness/inflexibility, alignment problems, growth spurt present, muscle strength imbalance, training method errors, poor footwear and training on hard surfaces. These factors are also described by Micheli and Klein (1991). One should question, how, whether the proposed person related risk factors are also present in non injured peers. The etiologic contribution of the growth spurt was, according to the authors, illustrated by the fact that in their retrospective analysis boys and girls showed a different pattern of traction apophysitis, according to the difference in the age of onset of the growth spurt. Proposed preventive measures included relative rest (e.g. the modification of sports activity in terms of frequency and magnitude of training), the prescription of non steroid anti inflammatory drugs, strength and flexibility training, supervised physiotherapy, etc.

Other measures proposed to prevent overuse injuries in children are: the use of padded protective devices (Meyers 1993), to match children according to age, maturity, skill, weight and height (matching for only the last two variables is considered practical) (Smith et al. 1993), to perform pre-participation examination to screen for rapid growth and the presence of other potential person-related risk factors (Smith et al. 1993) and to supervise all competitive sports (Smith et al. 1993). Furthermore it is advised to follow the 10% rule which indicates that in consecutive weeks the increase in the amount of training time, the amount of distance covered or the number of repititions performed in activity should not exceed 10% (Maffulli and Pintore 1990, Micheli and Klein 1991, Meyers 1993, Smith et al. 1993).

Common apophyseal injury sites

For the sake of clarity, some typical growth plate related injuries are mentioned in this paragraph since they can result in a growth disturbance, although it seems as if growth plate related overuse injuries in children are not very common and probably outnumbered by acute injuries.

Table 4. Examples of common apophyseal injury sites.

site	apophyseal injury
elbow	medial epicondyl apophysitis (Palmer's disease)
pelvis	iliac ischial apophysitis
knee	apophysitis of the inferior pole of the patella (Sinding Larsen Johansson syndrome) tibial tubercle apophysitis (Osgood Schlatter's disease)
foot	os calcis apophysitis (Sever's disease)

Both Micheli and Fehlandt (1992) and Gerrard (1993) give an overview of common apophyseal injury sites. It is beyond the scope of this review to discuss all these sites in depth. Examples are shown in table 4.

It should be kept in mind that when a child complains of persistent pain at any of these sites then apophysitis should be included in the diagnosis.

Conclusion

Children sustain both acute and overuse injuries, probably with an incidence that is lower than that of adults. It seems as if the majority of the injuries are of an acute nature, but it may well be that due to their self-limited nature, overuse injuries are by large under reported. Given the fact that much of the research suffers from methodological problems it is hard to give precise information. One can conclude that the risk of sustaining injuries is most likely closest linked with the type of sport and the quality and amount of exposure time. From the information available on the etiology of sports injuries of children it seems as if most of the injuries are avoidable, since many injuries contain a behavioral aspect. Prevention should therefore be focussed on a change of behaviour of the child, the parent, the teacher and the trainer or coach.

References

Backx FJG, Beijer HJM, Bol E and Erich. WBM Injuries in high-risk persons and high-risk sports. A longitudinal study of 1818 school children. The American Journal of Sports Medicine 19 (2): 124-130, 1991a.

Backx FJG. Sports injuries and youth. Etiology and prevention (doctoral thesis). University of Utrecht, the Netherlands, 1991b.

Backx FJG, Erich WBM, Kemper ABA and Verbeek ALM. Sports injuries in school-aged children. An epidemiologic study. The American Journal of Sports Medicine 17 (2): 234-240, 1989.

Baxter-Jones A., Maffulli N. and Helms P. Low injury rates in elite athletes. Archives of Disease in Childhood 68 130-132, 1993.

Bol E, Schmickli SL, Backx FJG, van Mechelen W. Sportblessures onder de knie; NISGZ publication 38, Papendal, 1991.

Chambers RB. Orthopedic injuries in athletes (ages 6- to 17), comparison of injuries occurring in six sports. Am. J. of Sp. Med. 7, 195-197, 1979.

de Loës M, K Goldi. Incidence rate of injuries during sport activity and physical exercise in a rural Swedish municipality: incidence rates in 17 sports. Int. J. Sports Med. 9: 461-467, 1988.

de Loës M. Epidemiology of sports injuries in the Swiss organization "Youth and Sports" 1987-1989. Int. J. of Sports Med. 16: 134-138, 1995.

Gerrard DF. Overuse injury and growing bones: the young athlete at risk. Br. J. Sports Mededicine 27 (1): 14-18, 1993.

Guyer B and Ellers B. Childhood Injuries in the United States. Mortality, Morbidity, and Cost. AJDC 144 649-652, 1990.

Hutson M. Community health, exercise and injury risk. Nursing Times aug.: 22-25, 1983.

Kaplan TA, Digel SL, Scavo VA, Arellana SB. Effect of obesity on injury risk in high school football players. Clinical J. of Sports Med. 5 (1): 43-47, 1995.

Klesges RC, Eck LH, Mellon MW, Fulliton W, Somes GW, Hanson CL. The accuracy of self-reports of physical activity. Med. and Sci. in Sports and Exerc. 22 (5): 690-697, 1990.

Kranenborg N. Sportbeoefening en blessures. T. Soc.. Gen. 60 (9): 224-227, 1982.

Linder MM, Towsend DJ, Jones JC, Balkom IL, Anthony CR. Incidence of adolescent injuries in junior high school football and its relation to sexual maturity. Clinical J. of Sports Med. 5 (3): 167-170, 1995.

Macera CA, Wooten W. Epidemiology of sports and recreation injuries among adolescents. Ped. Ex. Sci. 6: 424-433, 1994.

Maffulli N and Pintore E. Intensive training in young athletes. British Journal of Sports Medicine 24 (4): 237-239, 1990.

Maffulli N. The growing child in sport. Sports Medicine 48 (3): 561-568, 1992.

Mechelen W.v., Hlobil H, Kemper HCG. Incidence, Severity, Aetiology and Prevention of Sports Injuries. Sports Medicine 14 (2): 82-99, 1992.

Meyers JF. The Growing Athlete. In: Renström P.O. (Ed.), Sports Injuries: Basic Principles of Prevention and Care. Chapter 13: 178-193, Encyclopaedia of Sports Medicine Vol. IV, Blackwell Scientific Publications, Oxford, 1993.

Micheli LJ, Fehlandt AF. Overuse injuries to tendons and apophyses in children and adolescents. Clinics in Sports Medicine 11 (4): 713-726, 1992.

Micheli LJ, Klein JD. Sports injuries in children and adolescents. British Journal of Sports Medicine 25 (1): 6-9, 1991.

Shephard RJ. The Impact of Exercise upon Medical Costs. Sp. Med. 2: 133-143, 1985.

Smith AD, Andrish JT, Micheli LJ. The Prevention of Sport Injuries of Children and Adolescents. Medicine and Science in Sports and Exercise 25 (8): 1-7, 1993.

Stanitski CL. Management of Sports Injuries in Children and Adolescents. Orthopedic Clinics of North America 19 (4): 689-698, 1988.

Stanitski CL. Common injuries in preadolescent and adolescent children, Recommendations for intervention. Sports Med. 7 (1): 32-41, 1989.

Stuart MJ, Smith A. Injuries in junior A ice hockey. A three-year pospective study. Am. J. of Sports Medicine 23 (4):458-461, 1995.

Sturmans F. Epidemiologie. Dekker & van de Vegt (publ.), Nijmegen, 1984.

Tursz A, Crost M. Sports-related injuries in children. A study of their characteristics, frequency, and severity, with comparison to other types of accidental injuries. Am. J. of Sports Medicine 14 (4): 294-299, 1986.

van Galen W, Diederiks J. Sportblessures breed uitgemeten. Uitg. De Vrieseborch, Haarlem, 1990.

Walter SD, Sutton JR, McIntosh JM, Connolly C. The aetiology of sports injuries. A review of methodologies. Sports Med. 2: 47-58, 1985.

Watson A.W.S. Sports injuries during one academic year in 6799 Irish school children. The American Journal of Sports Medicine 12 (1): 65-71, 1984.

Zaricznyj B., Shattuck L.J.M., Mast T.A., Robertson R.V. and D'Elia G. Sports-related injuries in school-aged children. The American Journal of Sports Medicine 8 (5): 318-324, 1980.

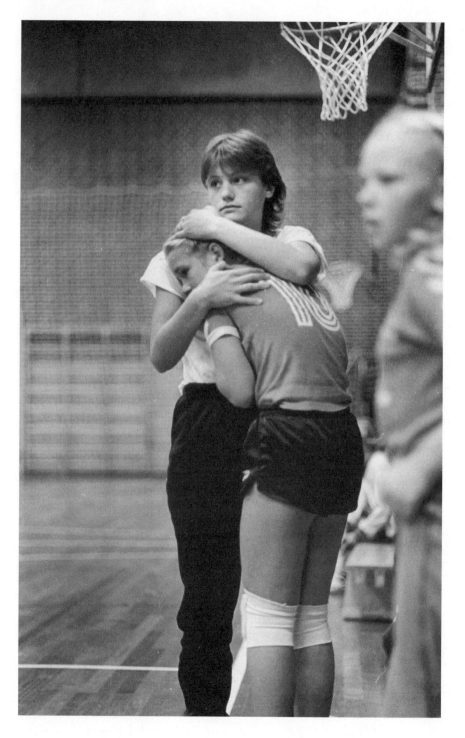

Chapter 16

Sport for Children and Youth Motivational Aspects

Yngvar Ommundsen

Organized sport for children and youth involves a large and important segment of contemporary Scandinavian societies. Sport participation within clubs is by far the most widespread and time consuming organized leisure time activity among Norwegian children and youth (Grue, 1985). Moreover, among Norwegian boys aged 11 to 15 on an average 60% are active sport club members and 57% report taking part in sports competitions (Wold, 1989). This pervasive interest for sport also seems to hold for other European countries (Patriksson, 1988; Campbell, 1986) as well as in the United States (Martens, 1986; Gould, 1987) and Australia (Robertson, 1986).

The paradox of sports for children and youth

Despite findings showing that young people are attracted to sport wherein competence may be demonstrated or enjoyment experienced (Kirshnit, Ham & Richards, 1989), research also show that young athletes drop out at strikingly high rates. Attrition rates have been found to be high both in American and European samples (Gould, 1987; Sack, 1977; Sisjord, 1993), and estimation rates show that generally 80% of those involved in sport drop out by the time they reach the age of 17 (Seefeldt, Blievernicht, Bruce & Gillian, 1978). Gould (1987), based on different studies of dropout prevalence, estimated that approximately 35% of those involved in youth sport discontinue involvement each year. Relatively high attrition rates have also been supported by Scandinavian studies (Patriksson, 1988; Skard & Vaglum, 1989). A particular decline in the number of participants has been found between the ages of 11 and 14 years of age (MMI, 1991; Roberts, 1984). In a prospective study among young Norwegian soccer players, aged 12 to 16 years, 22% dropped out during a period of 16 months (Ommundsen, 1992).

The socialization potential of sport for children and youth

It is generally believed that organized sport can enhance physical as well as psychosocial growth and development. Examples of potential effects attributed to sport include enhanced physical fitness and sport specific self-perception, the development of an active and healthy lifestyle. Moreover, several people have argued that sport promote social learning through internalization of culturally valued rules and norms and the value of acting prosocially (enculturation), development of positive relations to peers. Sport has also been regarded a vehicle with respect to structuring of social identity and safe exploration of personal capabilities. Finally, sport and exercise may be a resource for combating life stress (Gruber, 1985; Marsh, Richards & Barns, 1986; Kjørmo, 1988; Engstrøm, 1989; Wold, 1988; Horn, 1985; Coakley, 1987; Nilsson, 1988; Bredemeier & Shields, 1987; Estrada, Gelfand & Hartmann, 1988; Greendorfer, 1987; Kleiber & Richards, 1985; Brown & Siegel, 1988; Laging, 1981).

The nature of sport as a salient and highly valued achievement context, however, makes sport for children and youth a *double-edged sword*. On the one hand, sport may positively influence perceptions of competence and self-esteem, increase achievement expectancies and to lay the foundation for sustained sport interest and a physically active lifestyle. By contrast, stress, fear of failure, anxiety, the undermining of perceived competence and self-esteem, the reduction of subsequent achievement expectancies as well as reduced persistence in participation may also be the outcomes of sport involvement (Veroff, 1969; Roberts, 1981; Scanlan, 1984; Harter, 1985; Fox, 1987; Wankel & Sefton, 1989; Smith, 1986; Passer, 1988; Ommundsen, 1990).

The importance of motivational research

For valuable socialization outcomes to occur, young athletes have to enjoy sport, develop functional learning and motivational strategies and maintain their motivation for participating. It is believed that the sum of discrete, immediate experiences that children and youth are confronted with in sport, influences their feelings, moods and the perception of themselves in this context. In turn, the general emotional quality of the sport experience, has been found to be a powerful predictor of young peoples' sport motivation and persistence. Therefore, the study of the determinants of optimal sport motivation and persistence is essential in order to promote young peoples' attraction to sport, let them positively learn from sport and thereby produce beneficial physical and psychosocial outcomes.

Participation motivation and sport withdrawal

Why do several youngsters develop diminished motivation for sport and finally drop out? And why do some athletes develop dysfunctional motivational and achievement strategies when they participate in sport? Youth sport researchers have set out to understand why children and youth participate in sport and why they drop out. Investigations that have examined participation motives in children and youth sports reveal that young athletes value skill acquisition, having fun, playing for challenge, and becoming physically fit (Gill, Gross & Huddleston, 1985; Gould, Feltz & Weiss, 1985; Longhurst & Spink, 1987). Weiss and Petlichkoff (1989) concluded that the reasons can be categorized into four classifications: Competence, affilliation, fitness and fun. Moreover, these reasons seem to be universally accepted as the primary reasons for participation in sport. Although it seems that young athletes cite multiple reasons underlying their sport involvement, research suggests that comparing skills with others, personal accomplishments, improving skills and game excitement are the most important sources of enjoyment in children and youth sport (Wankel & Kreisel, 1985; Wankel & Sefton, 1989).

Athletes cite multiple reasons for dropping out of sport (Petlichkoff, 1993), but one might conclude that negative aspects of sport such as overemphasis on winning, did not make the team, lack of competence, competitive stress and dislike of coach contribute significantly to sport withdrawal (Gould & Petlichkoff, 1988).

Taken together, several studies on participation, motivation and sport withdrawal suggest that there is a mismatch between young peoples' expectations and motives for engaging in sport and situational and structional factors created within sport, leading to a negative view of their sport experience (Petlichkoff, 1993).

Despite the fact that such studies have increased our understanding of participation and withdrawal from sport, the focus of the literature has primarily been descriptive in nature. Theoretical models are needed that not only descibe the reasons young athletes cite for sport participation and withdrawal, but also set out to explain the cognitive and affective processes underlying these decisions. Adressing the need for theoretically based investigations, researchers have therefore started to test several motivational theories in the sport domain. A main aim has been to determine possible constructs and mechanisms underlying youngsters' motivational characteristics while participating in sport as well as their decision to further participate in or withdraw from sport.

Understanding the motivation of children and youth in sport

Generally organized sport for children and youth is comprised of structured competitive programs. Organized sport thus represents a classic achievement oriented context in which the individual or the team engage in mastery attempts striving to achieve a goal or standard of exellence and maximize performance. Moreover, organized sport for children and youth is usually a public affair. An adult led activity like this may be viewed as a competitive, challenging, socially evaluative achievement environment in which success is important, yet uncertain. All people involved, participants, parents, and coaches have a considerable amount of information on which to base their judgement about the young participant's sport competence. Organized sport for young people includes prevailing competitive norms, achievement related appraisals from significant others explicitly or implicitly communicated to the young participants. This fact, combined with the ability information derived from direct social comparison with teammates and opponents, make the potential for social evaluation in sport very high and the importance of being competent very salient (Scanlan, 1984; Veroff, 1969).

Recent theories of motivation have shown great potential in explaining variations in achievement related behavior and sport motivation (Duda, 1993; Weiss & Chaumeton, 1992). The most prevalent conceptual attempts to understand sport motivation have emerged out of contemporary motivational approaches that include social-cognitive theories of achievement motivation (Harter, 1978; Nicholls, 1984; Deci & Ryan, 1985). According to these theories, sets of cognitive and affective variables have motivational implications by mediating motivational aspects such as choice, effort and sport persistence. Both individual differences in cognitions and social contextual factors are assumed to have the potential to act as mediators between sport experiences and motivational outcomes. According to these theories, self-perceptions of competence seems to be the most important variable underlying subjective perception of success and failure (Duda, 1987). Moreover, the perception of demonstrated competence is ascribed a vital role in the initiation of motivated behavior within all these social cognitive theories of achievement motivation (Brustad, 1992).

The relevance of competence and achievement related theories in explaining motivation among children and youth in sport is further supported by research findings suggesting that children's attraction to sport is mainly based on the need for demonstrating competence. As previously mentioned, children very often cite competence related motives when asked why they participate in sport and enjoy sport. Second, results generally show that the average beginning age of participation in organized sport programmes ranges from 7 to 12 years of age (Passer, 1988). This is an age range in which children typically seem to reach a cognitive stage of development by which they develop the ability to make use of social comparison information in the establishment of standards for evaluating the goodness of their own performance (France-Kaatrude & Smith, 1985). In order to socially compare their abilities, therefore, children from 6 and 7 years old often begin to transform all sorts of situations into competitive ones (Veroff, 1969; Ruble, Boggiano, Feldman & Loebl, 1980; Ommundsen, 1991). Similarly, research from sport and physical game situations reveals that competition becomes an independent social motive around the age of 7. Studies also indicate that children from various countries will increase their competitive behavior when social comparison information is made available (Toda, Shinotsuka, Mc Clintock & Stech, 1978).

Motivational theories related to competence and achievement

According to Harter's **competence motivation theory**, young people are intrinsically motivated to deal effectively with the environment, and they do so by engaging in mastery attempts (White, 1959; Harter, 1978). In a similar vein, Nicholls (1984) **achievement goal theory** holds that the feeling of competence is the major goal of achievement behavior. Consequently, individuals will behave in a manner to maximize the demonstration of high ability and minimize the demonstration of low ability (Nicholls, 1984). The major tenet of **cognitive evaluation theory** (Deci & Ryan, 1985) is that intrinsic motivation is maximized when individuals feel competent and self-determining in dealing with their environment.

Although these theoretical approaches clearly focus upon partly different motivational aspects and mechanisms, they have several features in common. In particular this holds for Nicholls' achievement goal theory and Deci & Ryan's cognitive evaluation theory. Accordingly, efforts have been made to bridge the gap between these two approaches to motivation (Butler, 1988; Deci & Ryan, 1989; Duda et al, 1995; Thill & Brunel, 1995).

In the following, Harter's competence motivation theory and Nicholls' achievement goal theory will be outlined in more detail together with a presentation of relevant empirical studies. These two theoretical approaches have been extensively examined within the domain of sport for children and youth (see Duda, 1993a; Weiss & Chaumeton, 1992 and Weiss, 1987 for a review) and seems valuable in order to understand motivational aspects of sport for children and youth.

Competence motivation theory

Harter's conceptual model depicts perceived social approval, perceived competence, an internal sense of personal control and affect as factors that directly and/or indirectly influence motivation. Perceived competence and affect are key constructs in competence motivation theory along with the role of significant others on young peoples' developing self-preceptions of competence and control (Harter, 1978; 1980; 1981a). According to Harter, parents and coaches play an important role in shaping children's emerging perceptions of competence and control through the type of evaluative feedback that they provide in response to the young athlete's achievement efforts. Specifically, an individual who perceives positive approval from significant others and who has high perceptions of competence and internal control in domains where the individual values competence will experience increased self-worth, which will result in positive emotions, and subsequently, increased intrinsically motivated behavior.

According to this theory, successful mastery attempts with optimal challenges and positive reactions from significant others will increase an individual's motivation to again approach achievement tasks (Harter & Connell, 1984). Such an increase in motivation is hypothezied to be mediated by increased intrinsic motivational orientation (Harter, 1981b), higher perceptions of competence and internal control, and enhanced positive affect. In addition, successful mastery attempts are also assumed to develop the use of internal criteria and mastery goals to evaluate success and guide judgements about level of competence.

By contrast, unsuccessful mastery attempts followed by negative reactions from significant others will produce decreased perceived competence, an external locus of control, increase the use of external criteria to evaluate performance outcomes and will depend upon external standards to guide the evaluation of levels of competence. Subsequently, the result is increased levels of anxiety in mastery situations as well as a greater possibility that further mastery attempts are avoided.

Empirical studies based on competence motivation theory

Weiss et al (1990) examined the relationship between young athletes' perceptions of competence and their attributions for performance success in the sport domain. Results revealed that children high in perceived competence made attributions that were more internal and stable and higher in personal control than their low-perceived-competence peers. Thus, children with positive self-perceptions of ability adopted a more intrinsic orientation to explain their performance ratings; and these attributional patterns are likely to lead to positive affect, future success expectations and continued sport motivation. In support for this supposition, Ommundsen and Vaglum (1991), in a study among young soccer players, found that high perceived soccer competence was associated with higher levels of enjoyment in soccer, whereas low soccer-specific self-esteem was related to higher levels of soccer competition anxiety. Burton & Martens (1986) found that young dropouts from wrestling exibited lower perceived wrestling competence than those still involved. Parallel findings where obtained in a study among interscholastic sport participants (Feltz & Petlichkoff, 1983). Klint (1988) found that among young female gymnasts, high levels of enjoyment and perceived competence both were strong contributors to scores on choice, effort and persistence as measures of motivation.

Petlichkoff (1993) prospectively examined group differences among interscholastic sport participants on perceived ability and satisfaction in sport by means of three assessments over the course of a sport season. The groups consisted of starters (those who generally played from the start of the game), non-starters (those who were the first players off the bench) and survivors (those who sat on the bench most of the time). Results showed that sitting on the bench most of the time negatively influenced survivors' sport satisfaction over the course of the season. Moreover, survivors showed the lowest ratings on self-perception of sport competence at all three assessments. These results indicate that sport situations in which some children are not allowed to demonstrate their competence and obtain successfull mastery attempts, negatively influence their perceived ability and enjoyment in sport. This group who may very well consist of late matures (Barnsley & Thomson, 1988; Petlichkoff, 1993) may easily become next year's dropouts (Weiss & Petlichkoff, 1989). Therefore any attempt should be made to meet the needs of each individual in sport programs, regardless of his or her present ability.

Black and Weiss (1991) were interested in the influence of significant others' behavior on self-perceptions of ability among young competitive swimmers. Contingent praise and information from coaches following successful performances and contingent encouragement and corrective information following performance errors were associated with athletes who were higher in perceived success and competence as well as higher in their enjoyment of the sport and preference for optimal challenges. Supporting these results Brustad (1993) found that children who reported that their parents consistently responded with support and encouragement for their sport-related efforts displayed greater intrinsic motivation, in the form of higher preference for challenge, than did their counterparts who received less favourable parental support. Studies conducted among young Norwegian soccer players and young American basketball and tennis players have shown a similar pattern of results (Ommundsen & Vaglum, 1991; Brustad, 1988; Leff & Hoyle, 1995). Other studies (Felson & Reed, 1986) have shown that the positive relationship between parental judgement of children's athletic abilities and the child's self-appraisals holds even when levels of actual child ability were statistically controlled.

In sum, sufficient perceived sport competence seems to be an important precursor of positive affect and sustained motivation in sport among children and youth. Results also suggest that significant others have an important role in shaping young athletes' self-perception characteristics. In particular, providing encouragement, positive reinforcement and corrective feedback seems to enhance young peoples' self-perceptions in sport. It should be emphasized, however, that the quantity of reinforcement and the mere use of positive statements are not sufficient to influence changes in perceived competence (Horn, 1985). Rather, as Weiss (1993) has underscored: "It is the quality of significant others' behaviors, specifically the contingency to athletes' behavior and the appropriateness of the information given, that is crucial to young athletes' cognitions about the meaning of these messages".

Achievement goal theory

One central assumption of achievement goal theory is that variations in motivational goal perspectives are a crucial dimension influencing variations in motivation. In particular, it is assumed that an individual's goal perspective impacts on how that person cognitively interprets, affectively responds to, and behaves in achievement-related settings (Nicholls, 1984; Nicholls, 1989; Duda, 1992; Dweck, 1986). As opposed to Harter's competence motivation theory (Harter, 1978), achievement goal theory is less concerned with how much competence an individual perceives, and focuses more on conceptions of competence, that is how competence or ability is subjectively constructed (Nicholls, 1984; Duda, 1987).

Two distinct goal perspectives are presumed to be operating in achievement environments, namely task involvement and ego involvement. These two goals are assumed to relate to how an individual subjectively evaluates his or her level of competence within sport. When children are task involved, the experience of learning, personal improvement and/or meeting the demands of the task generate feelings of competence and success. In this case, the perception of own ability is self-referenced. In ego involvement on the other hand, beating others and demonstrating superior ability are bases for subjective success. Much concern is centered around not showing that one is less able than others when ego-involved. This is because perceptions of competence are normatively or other-referenced when a person has adopted an ego-involved goal perspective (Elliott & Dweck, 1988).

The motivational implications of goal perspectives
Achievement goal theory would hypothesize that functional motivated behavior will be demonstrated by task involved young athletes who judge ability in self-referent terms, irrespective of each individual's level of perceived competence. Functional motivated behavior includes the selection of achievement strategies

such as exerting effort, choosing tasks that are moderately challenging, continued motivation and persistence when experiencing unsuccessfull mastery attempts (Dweck & Leggett, 1988; Elliott & Dweck, 1988).

In contrast, ego-oriented individuals who define competence in norm-referenced terms, will exibit functional motivated behavior if they have high perceptions of competence. They are presumed to show dysfunctional motivated behavior if perceptions of competence are low. Any lack of demonstrated competence relative to others then becomes a threat to their self-esteem (de Charms, 1972) and will induce stress (Lazarus & Folkman, 1984). Dysfunctional motivated behavior among this group of athletes would include such categories as reduced effort or cease to try in the face of difficulty or failure, and choosing easy or hard tasks to avoid challenge. Performance impairment and dropping out are also assumed to be the consequences of ego involvement when the adequacy of one's ability is in doubt (Dweck & Leggett, 1988).

All these dysfunctional motivated behaviors may be looked upon as strategies used to save face and protect their self-esteem in public image threathening situations (Covington & Omelich, 1979; Snyder et al, 1976). It has been the contention of several researchers (Horn & Hasbrook, 1986; Roberts, 1986) that there will be an increase in anxiety, perceptions of stress and dropout from sport for youngsters as they increase their focus on relative ability.

Developmental factors influencing achievement goals

According to Nicholls (1978, 1984; Nicholls & Miller, 1984ab), young children do not, however, differentiate between the concepts of ability and effort until after the age of 12. Thus children below 12 years of age do not show signs of ego goal involvement and are therefore less likely to demonstrate dysfunctional motivated behavior, like for example dropping out of sport (Roberts, 1984). This line of reasoning corresponds to age specific dropout prevalences found in several studies previously mentioned, showing that dropout rates are accelerated after 11 to 12 years of age. For ego involvement to occur in children, they must be able to assess the relative effect of effort and ability to success and failure in sport (Whitehead & Dalby, 1987). It is first when the concepts of ability and effort are differentiated from each other, and ability is conceived as a capacity that one is able to understand, that one's ability limits the effect that additional effort can have on increased performance (Nicholls, 1984; Duda, 1987; Stipek & McIver, 1989). Nicholls proposes that once the conception of ability as capacity has been attained by a person, he or she will be able to utilize either the differentiated (i.e. ego involved) or undifferentiated (i.e. task involved) conception of ability.

Situational/contextual factors influencing achievement goals

The probability of invoking task involvement or ego involvement is also dependent upon contextual factors and situational cues (Ames, 1992; Nicholls, 1989). The goal perspectives of children and youth sport participants are hypothesized to be adopted through an interplay with the social environment over time. Preferences for task or ego involved goals are presumed to develop through repeated interactions with significant others such as parents and coaches. In particular, situations that emphasize interpersonal competition, public evaluation and a reward structure comprising normative feedback, are likely to invoke social comparison processes in young athletes. Social comparison in turn elicits the use of the differentiated conception of ability and individuals become ego involved. Alternatively, in situations in which coaches emphasize the learning process, effort, improvement and skill development, task goals are more likely to emerge (Ames, 1992). A varied and diversed task structure and a high degree of participation in decision-making among athletes are also regarded as important aspects of a task involving motivational climate (Rosenholtz & Simpson, 1984).

Parents and coaches make their goal preferences clear when they talk to the children about his or her activities. By giving certain cues, and rewards and making explicit expectations, these significant others may structure the motivational climate in such a way that it makes one conception of ability or the other manifest (Roberts, 1992b).

Empirical studies based on achievement goal theory

Correlates of achievement goals
There is evidence that achievement goals do function in sport. Research has been directed at developing measures of task and ego goals, investigating the behavioral, cognitive and affective correlates of goal perspectives in sport, and investigating the impact of goal perspectives on young athletes' motivation and achievement strategies (Duda, 1993).

One of the most consistent findings in the goal perspective literature is the observed link between task involvement and reported enjoyment of, and interest in sport among young participants (Duda, 1993b). Regardless of competence level and competitive outcome, task orientation positively relates to enjoyment and interest (Duda, 1993; Duda et al, 1992). In a study among young sport participants, Duda and co-workers (Duda, 1993b), found that a high task orientation, as opposed to a high ego orientation, was coupled with greater investment and persistence in the competitive sport experience. In line with these results, Ewing (1981) among her sample of young current and former athletes found that those who were focused on ego involvement were more likely to have ceased their involvement in sport. Weitzer (1989) found that boys and girls who emphasized task goals in sport, regardless of their actual ability, participated in sports and physical activities more than did boys and girls who strongly endorsed ego involved goals.

Taken together, these results support predictions stemmed from goal perspective theory, and suggest that young athletes who are ego involved and doubt their ability, may develop motivational difficulties and give up sport or not even try sport at all. Young athletes under age 11 or 12 years, however, do not seem to have an ego involved goal perspective (Roberts & Treasure,1992) and are, therefore, more unlikely to develop motivational deficits leading to dropout.

Other studies have investigated the relationship of goal perspectives to beliefs about the causes of sport success and achievement strategies in sport. Task involved athletes seems to endorse the view that hard work, effort and persistence are the causes of achievement and learning in sport, whereas those ego involved believe that ability and talent alone account for variations in sport success (Hom et al, 1993; Duda et.al., 1992; Boyd & Callaghan, 1994; Treasure & Roberts, 1994). Individuals have much to gain from believing that success in sport is achieved through hard work, a factor that is clearly within their control.

Task involved participants also seem to be more apt to report the use of adaptive achievement strategies in competition and practice such as liking practice and taking additional practice (Lochbaum & Roberts, 1993; Roberts & Ommundsen, 1996). Clearly, holding the belief that effort and persistence is the cause of learning and achievement, and using adaptive achievement strategies reflects a more functional motivational pattern.

Studies have also attempted to examine the linkage between the self-reported achievement goals of parents and these goals as perceived by the children, and corresponding personal achievement goals of the children in sport. Duda & Hom (1993) and Ebbeck and Becker (1994) found that young soccer and basketball players who were higher in task involvement perceived their parents to be higher in task involvement. The same held for ego involvement. No significant relationship was found, however, between players' goal perspectives and the actual self-reported goal perspectives of parents (Duda & Hom, 1993). Therefore, parents appear to play a role as a socializing agent in terms of children's goal perspectives in sport, but this influence seems to be an indirect one, mediated by individual player perceptions.

Piparo et al (cited in Duda, 1993), examined young athletes' perceptions of their coaches' behaviors as potential predictors of their achievement goal perspectives. Results indicated that greater coach encouragement related to a stronger focus on task goals, whereas greater perceived coach use of a pressuring style was a significant and negative predictor of task goals among the young athletes.

Correlates of the situational goal structure
Walling et al, (1993) investigated correlates of the situational goal structure or perceived motivational climate among young athletes and found that perceptions of a task-involving goal structure were positively related to satisfaction with being a team member and negatively associated with performance worry in competitions. The reverse was true for perceptions of an ego-involving goal structure. Ommundsen et al, (1995) examined the relationship between perceived situational goal structures and achievement strategies among team sport members and found that these constructs were related in a conceptually meaningfull manner. Perception of the team sport goal structure as task oriented corresponded to self-reported use of functional achievement strategies, including elements of motivation such as persistence in practice.

Thill & Brunell (1995) experimentally induced a task involving, and an ego involving situational goal structure among two samples of young soccer players, aged 6 to 10 and 11 to 15, respectively, in order to examine whether people mobilize different conceptions of ability or achievement goals when manipulating the situational goal structure. Based on self-reports of effort on a penalty shot task, the results indicate that in sport settings, children from 6 to 10 years of age use the less differentiated conception of ability in both task and ego involving conditions. By contrast, the athletes between 11 and 15 years of age tend to use the differentiated conception of ability when faced with an ego involving situational goal structure. These results support the developmental aspects of goal perspectives theory, and suggest that among young athletes below 11 years of age, the induction of ego involving situational goal structures do not negatively affect motivation such as withdrawal of effort, whereas it does so among older groups.

Treasure & Roberts (1995) manipulated the situational goal structure among groups of sixth and seventh grade children within the context of school sport, and found that subjects in the task treatment group preferred to engage in challenging tasks, believed success was the result of motivation and effort, and experienced more satisfaction with the activity than subjects in the ego treatment condition.

A very significant finding from this study is the fact that by manipulating specific structures of the achievement context, such as reward and evaluation procedures, grouping of children, design of tasks and activities, and involving children in decision making processes, sport practitioners can affect the situational goal structure towards a task orientation. The impact of manipulating the goal structure towards task involvement may even be so powerful that it overrides existing ego-involving achievement goals of the young participants.

In summary, a task oriented motivational climate or goal structure seems to have positive motivational consequences, whereas inducing an ego involving situational goal structure may be emotionally and motivationally detrimental. In particular this may be the case after the age of 11, when children seems capable of making use of either a task oriented achievement goal (i.e., the undifferentiated conception of ability) or an ego oriented achievement goal (i.e., the differentiated conception of ability).

Research further suggests that significant others may influence the situational goal structure or the kind of motivational climate youngsters perceive in sport. By means of their way of behaving and communicating, parents and coaches may positively or negatively influence young athletes' affective sport experiences, their motivational strategies and their sustained motivation in sport. Results also suggest that the situational goal structure or motivational climate is dynamic in nature and may be altered through intervention efforts.

Recommendations for practice

* To increase enjoyment levels in sport should be regarded an important task, both in its own right and because high enjoyment seems to enhance intrinsic motivation and prevent young sport participants from dropping out. In order to increase enjoyment levels among young athletes, it seems essential to enhance their sense of competence in sport. This can be done by maximizing the opportunities for participation for all, and by matching the difficulty of sport skills and goals to the developmental capabilities of the participants.

* Adults involved in sport programs for children and youth must ensure high quality in the interactions children have with significant others such as parents, and coaches as well as peers. It is imperative that adults become aware of the role they play in the development of perceived competence in young athletes, and that they structure their performance feedback and general communication styles to enhance youngsters' perceptions of ability and sport motivation.

* To help children who underestimate their perceived competence, adults may encourage them to make unstable but controllable attributions of their own "failures" in sport, such as lack of effort, and wrong strategy. This may enhance perceived competence and sport motivation. Appropriate goal setting and giving contingent feedback may also help reverse a spiral of negative evaluations and ensuing unmotivated behavior.

* Promoting functional causal explanations among young athletes for less successful mastery attempts, may also prove effective to reduce sport competition anxiety and dropout.

* Adults involved in sport programs should also emphasize the development of a task oriented conception of ability among young sport participants. Parents should be made aware of the influence of their own achievement goals upon the goals of the young athlete, and they should be encouraged to define sport success in a self-referenced manner. This may help young athletes develop a task oriented goal perspective.

* Coaches should create a task involving situational goal structure among young athletes. The sport environment should be structured in a task focused manner such that learning and development becomes salient, not performance or normative references outcomes. Then, motivation and enjoyment among all participants will be enhanced, not just those who perceive themselves to be high in relative ability.

* Sport organizers should also be aware of the the institutional value structure that characterizes children and youth sport associations. As suggested by Lee (Lee, 1995), the prevailing value system may influence situational goal structure that adults within each particular sports group choose to emphasize. Consequently, it may be easier for parents and coaches to create a task oriented situational goal structure in their own sport groups, if the total institutional value structure in which they are embedded also reflect a task involved philosophy of sport.

I will conclude by arguing that more young athletes may sustain their sport motivation if they are reinforced to do their best rather than be the best.

References

Ames, C (1984). Competitive, cooperative and individualistic goal structures: A cognitive-motivational analysis. In: Ames, R & Ames, C (Eds.). Research on motivation in education. Vol.1: Student motivation. pp.177-208. New York: Academic Press.

Ames, C (1992). The relationship of achievement goals to student motivation in classroom settings. In: Roberts, GC (Ed.). Motivation in sport and exercise. Champaign, Illinois: Human Kinetics.

Ames, C & Archer, J (1988). Achievement goals in the classroom: Students' learning strategies and motivation processes. J of Educational Psychology, 80, 260-267.

Barnsley, RH & Thompson, AH (1988). Birthdate and success in minor hockey: The key to the NHL. Canadian J of Behavioral Science, 20, 167-176.

Boyd, M & Callaghan, J (1994). Task and ego goal perspectives in organized youth sport. International J of Sport Psychology,22, 411-424.

Bredemeier, BJ & Shields, DL (1987). Moral growth through physical activity: A structural/develpomental approach. In: Gould, D & Weiss, MR (Eds.). Advances in sport pediatrics, vol. 2, behavioral issues. pp. 43-60. Champaign, Illinois: Human Kinetics.

Brown JD, Siegel JM (1988). Exercise as a buffer of life stress: A prospective study of adolescent health. Health Psychology, 7, 341-353.

Brustad, RJ (1988). Affective outcomes in competitive youth sport: The influence of intrapersonal and socialization factors. J of Sport Psychology, 10, 307-321.

Brustad, RJ (1992). Integrating socialization influences into the study of children's motivation in sport. J of Sport & Exercise Psychology,14, 59-77

Burton, D & Martens, R (1986). Pinned by their own goals: An exploratory investigation into why kids drop out of wrestling. J of Sport Psychology, 8, 183-197.

Butler, R (1988). Enhancing and undermining intrinsic motivation: The effects of task-involving and ego-involving evaluation on interest and performance. British J of Educational Psychology, 58, 1-14.

de Charms, R (1972). Personal causation training in the schools. J of Applied Social Psychology, 2, 95-113.

Campbell, S (1986). Youth sport in the United Kingdom. In: Weiss, M & Gould, D (Eds). Sport for children and youth. The 1984 Olympic Scientific Congress Proceedings vol, 10 pp 21-26. Champaign Illinois: Human Kinetics.

Coakley, JJ (1987). Children and the sport socialization process. In: Gould, D & Weiss, MR (Eds.). Advances in sport pediatrics, vol. 2, behavioral issues. pp. 43-60. Champaign, Illinois: Human Kinetics.

Covington, MV (1984). The self-worth theory of achievement motivation: Findings and implications. The Elementary School Journal, 85, 5-20.

Covington, MV & Omelich, CL (1979). Effort: the double-edged sword in school achievement. J of Educational Psychology, 71, 169-182.

Deci, EL & Ryan, RM (1985). Intrinsic motivation and self-determination in human behavior. New York: Plenum.

Duda, JL (1987). Towards a developmental theory of childrens motivation in sport. J of Sport Psychology, 9, 130-145.

Duda J (1988). The relationship between goal perspectives, persistence and behavioral intensity among male and female recreational sport participants. Leisure Sciences, 10, 95-106.

Duda, J (1989). Goal perspectives, participation and persistence in sport. International J of Sport Psychology, 20, 42-56.

Duda, J (1992). Motivation in sport settings: A goal persepctive approach. In: Roberts, GC (Ed.). Motivation in sport and exercise. Champaign, Illinois: Human Kinetics.

Duda, JL (1993). Goals: a social cognitive approach to the study of achievement motivation in sport. In: Singer, RN, Murphey, M & Tennant, LK (Eds). Handbook of research on sport psychology. NY: McMillan publishing Company. (pp. 421-466).

Duda, JL (1993). The development of children's motivation: A goal perspective approach. In: Developmental issues in children's sport and physical education. Whitehead, J (Ed). Bedford college of higher education, Bedford, UK.

Duda, JL, Fox, K, Biddle, SJH & Armstrong, N (1992). Children's achievement goals and beliefs about success in sport. British J of Educational Psychology, 62, 313-423.

Duda, JL & Hom Jr. (1993). Inter-dependencies between the perceived and self-reported goal orientations of young athletes and their parents. Pediatric exercise Science,5, 234-241.

Duda, JL, Chi, L, Newton, ML, Walling, MD & Catley, D (1995). Task and ego orientation and intrinsic motivation in sport. International J of Sport Psychology, 26, 40-63.

Dweck, CS (1986). Motivational processes affecting learning. American Psychologist, 41, 1040-48.

Dweck CS, Leggett EL (1988). A social cognitive approach to motivation and personality. Psychological Review, 95, 256-273.

Ebbeck, V & Becker, SL (1994). Psychosocial predictors of goal orientations in sport. Research Q for Exercise & Sport, 65, 355-362.

Elliott, ES and Dweck, CS (1988). Goals: An approach to motivation and achievement. J of Personality and Social Psychology, 54, 5-12.

Ewing, ME (1981). Achievement orientations and sport behavior of males and females. Unpublished doctoral dissertation, University of Illinois at Urbana-Champaign.

Felson, RB & Reed, M (1986). The effect of parents on the self-appraisals of children. Social Psychology Quarterly, 49, 302-308.

Feltz, DL and Petlichkoff, L (1983). Perceived competence among interscholastic sport participants and drop-outs. Canadian J of Applied Sport Sciences, 8, 231-235.

France-Kaatrude, AC & Smith,WP (1985). Social comparison, task motivation, and the develpoment of self-evaluative standards in children. Developmental Psychology, 21, 1080-89.

Gill, DL, Gross, JB & Huddleston, S (1983). Participation motivation in youth sports. International J of Sport Psychology, 14, 1-14.

Gould D, Feltz DL, Horn TS, Weiss MR (1982). Reasons for attrition in competitive youth swimming. J of Sport Behavior, 5, 135-165.

Gould, D & Horn, T (1984). Participation motivation in young athletes. In: Silva, JM & Weinberg,RS (Eds.). Psychological foundations of sport. pp. 359-370. Champaign, Illinois: Human Kinetics.

Gould D, Feltz D, Weiss MR (1985). Motives for participating in competitive youth swimming. International Journal of Sport Psychology, 16, 126-140.

Gould, D (1987). Understanding attrition in children's sport.In D. Gould & M. Weiss (Eds.). Advances in pediatric sport sciences-behavioral issues (pp. 61-85). Champaign Illinois: Human Kinetics.

Gould, D & Petlichkoff, L (1988). Participation motivation and attrition in young athletes. In: Smoll, F.L., Magill, R.A. & Ash, M.J. (Eds.), Children in Sport pp.161-178. Champaign IL: Human Kinetics.

Greendorfer, S (1987). Psychosocial correlates of organized physical activity. J of Physical Education, Recreation & Dance, 11, 59-64.

Gruber, JJ (1985). Physical activity and self-esteem development in children: A meta analysis. American Academy of Physical Education Papers, 19, 30-48.

Grue, L (1985). Bedre enn sitt rykte. En undersøkelse av ungdoms fritidsbruk (Not so black as they are painted. An investigation into young peoples' use of their leisure time). Oslo: STUI.

Harter, S (1978). Effectance motivation reconsidered. Human development, 21, 34-64.

Harter, S (1980). The development of competence motivation in the mastery of cognitive and physical skills: Is there still a place for joy? In: Roberts, G.C. and Landers, D.M. (Eds.). Psychology of motor behavior and sport. Illinois: Human Kinetics Publishers.

Harter, S (1981a). A model of mastery motivation in children: Individual differences and developmental change. In: Collins, A (Ed.). Minnesota symposium on child psychology Vol. 14, 215-255. Hillsdale, NJ:Erlbaum

Harter, S (1981b). A new self-report scale of intrinsic versus extrinsic motivation in the classroom. Developmental Psychology, 17, 300-312.

Harter, S. & Connell, J (1984). A model of childrens achievement and related self-perceptions of competence, control and motivational orientation. In: Nicholls, J (Ed.). The development of achievement motivation. Greenwich, CT: JAI Press.

Hom Jr, LH, Duda, JL & Miller, A (1993). Correlates of goal orientations among young athletes. Pediatric Exercise Science,5, 168-176.

Horn, TS (1985). Coaches' feedback and changes in children's perceptions of their physical competence. J of Educational Psychology, 77, 174-186.

Horn, TS (1987). The influence of teacher-coach behavior on the psychological development of children. In: Gould, D & Weiss, MR (Eds.). Advances in sport pediatrics, vol. 2, behavioral issues. pp. 121-142. Champaign, Illinois: Human Kinetics.

Horn, TS & Hasbrook, C (1986). Informational components influencing children's perceptions of their physical competence. In: Weiss, M & Gould, D (Eds). Sport for children and youth. The 1984 Olympic Scientific Congress Proceedings vol, 10 pp. 81-88. Champaign Illinois: Human Kinetics.

Kirshnit, CE, Ham, M & Richards, MH (1989). The sporting life: Athletic activities during early adolescence. Journal of Youth and Adolescence, 18, 601-615.

Klint, K & Weiss, MR (1986). Dropping in and dropping out: Participation motives of current and former youth gymnasts.Canadian J of Applied Sport Sciences, 11, 106-114.

Klint, KA & Weiss, MR (1987). Perceived competence and motives for participating in youth sports: A test of Harters competence motivation theory. J of Sport Psychology, 9, 55-65.

Laging, R (1981). Ein didaktisches modell zum soziales Lernen. Sportunterricht, 30, 464-472.

Lazarus, RS & Folkman, S (1984). Stress, appraisal, and coping. New York: Springer.

Lee, MJ (1995). Relationship between values and motives in sport. In: Proceedings part 2. IXth European congress on sport psychology (Vanfraechem – Raway, R & Vanden Welden, Y (Eds). Belgian federation of sport psychology. (pp. 681-688).

Leff, SS & Hoyle, RH (1995). Young athletes' perceptions of parental support and pressure. J of Youth and Adolescence, 24, 187-203.

Lochbaum, MR & Roberts, GC (1993). Goal orientations and perceptions of the sport experience. J of Sport & Exercise Psychology, 15, 160-171.

Markeds-og mediainstituttet (1991). Barne- og ungdomsundersøkelsen (The children and youth study). Oslo: Markeds- og mediainstituttet.

Marsh, HW, Richards, GE and Barnes, J (1986). Multidimensional self-concepts: The effect of participation in an outward bound program. J of Personality and Social Psychology, 50, 195-204.

Martens, R (1986). Youth sport in the United States. In: Weiss, M & Gould, D (Eds.). Sport for children and youth. The 1984 Olympic Scientific Congress Proceedings vol.10 pp 27-33. Champaign Illinois: Human Kinetics.

Nicholls, JG (1984). Striving to demonstrate and develop ability: A theory of achievement motivation. In: Nicholls, JG (Ed.). The development of achievement motivation. Greenwich, CT: JAI Press.

Nicholls, JG (1989). The competitive ethos and democratic education. Cambridge, Mass.: Harvard University Press.

Nicholls, JG & Miller, A (1984a). Conceptions of ability and achievement motivation. In Ames, R. & Ames, C. (Eds.). Research on Motivation in education: Student motivation. Volume 1. pp. 39-73. NY: Academic Press.

Nicholls, J and Miller, A (1984b). Development and its discontents: the differentiation of the concept of ability. In: Nicholls, J (eds): Advances in motivation and achievement. A research annual. pp. 185-218. Greenwich, Connecticut: JAI Press Inc.

Ommundsen, Y (1990). Barn og konkurranseidrett i et psykologisk perspektiv (Children and competitive sport: A psychological perspective). Barn, 8, 73-88.

Ommundsen, Y (1991). Når bør barn begynne med idrettskonkurranser? En teoretisk drøfting samt enkelte forslag til retningslinjer for konkurranseoppstart (Competitive readiness in children: A theoretical discussion and some directions concerning initial involvement in competitions). Barn, 9, 36-50.

Ommundsen, Y & Vaglum, P (1991). Soccer competetion anxiety and enjoyment in young boy players. The influence of perceived competence and significant others'emotional involvement. International J of Sport Psychology,22, 35-49.

Ommundsen, Y & Vaglum, P (1992). Sport-specific influences: Impact on persistence in soccer among adolescent antisocial soccer players. J of Adolescent Research, 4, 507-521.

Ommundsen, Y (1992). Self-evaluation, affect and dropout in the soccer domain: A prospective study of young male Norwegian players. The Norwegian University for Sport & Physical Education, Oslo. Doctoral thesis.

Ommundsen, Y, Roberts, GC & Kavussanu, M (1996). Perceived motivational climate and cognitive and affective correlates among team sport athletes. Journal of Sport Sciences (submitted).

Passer, M.W. (1988). Determinants and consequences of children's competitive stress. In: Smoll, F.L., Magill, R.A. & Ash, M.J. (Eds.). Children in Sport (pp. 203-227). Champaign IL: Human Kinetics.

Patriksson, G. (1988). Theoretical and empirical analyses of drop-out from youth sports in Sweden. Scandinavian J of Sports Sciences, 10, 29-37.

Petlichkoff, LM (1993). Group differences on achievement goal orientations, perceived ability, and level of satisfaction during an athletic season. Pediatric Exercise Science, 5, 12-24.

Roberts, GC, Kleiber, DA and Duda, JL (1981). An analysis of motivation in childrens' sport: The role of perceived competence in participation. J of Sport Psychology, 3, 206-216.

Roberts, G.C. (1984). Achievement motivation in childrens' sport. In Nicholls, J.G. (Ed.). Advances in motivation and achievement pp. 251-281. Greenwich Connecticut: JAI Press

Roberts, GC (1986). The perception of stress: A potential source and its development. In: Weiss, M & Gould, D (Eds.). Sport for children and youth. The 1984 Olympic Scientific Congress Proceedings vol.10 pp 119-126. Champaign Illinois: Human Kinetics.

Roberts, GC & Treasure, DC (1992). Children in sport. Sport Science Review, 1, 46-64.

Roberts, GC & Ommundsen, Y (1996). Effect of goal orientations on achievement beliefs, cognitions and strategies. Scandinavian J of Medicine & Science in Sports, 6, 46-56.

Robertson, I (1986). Youth sport in Australia. In: Weiss, M & Gould, D (Eds). Sport for children and youth. The 1984 Olympic Scientific Congress Proceedings vol.10. pp 5-10. Champaign Illinois: Human Kinetics.

Robinson, TT & Carron, AV (1982). Personal and situational factors associated with dropping out versus maintaining participation in competitive sport. Journal of Sport Psychology 4, 364-378.

Ruble, DN, Boggiano, AK, Feldman, NS & Loebl, JH (1980). A developmental analysis of the role of social comparison in self-evaluation. Developmental Psychology, 16, 105-115.

Ryan, RM & Deci, EL (1989). Bridging the research traditions of task/ego involvement and intrinsic/extrinsic motivation: Comment of Butler (1987). J of Educational Psychology, 81, 265-268.

Sack, HG (1977). Der Austritt Jugendlicher-einige von vielen hintergrunden. Olympische Jugend, 12, (3) 12-16.

Scanlan, TK (1988). Social evaluation and the competition process: A developmental perspective. In Smoll, FL, Magill, RA & Ash, MJ (Eds.), Children in Sport (pp. 135-148). Champaign IL: Human Kinetics.

Scanlan, TK & Lewthwaite, R (1986). Social psychological aspects of competition for male youth sport participants: 4 Predictors of enjoyment. J of Sport Psychology, 8, 25-35.

Seefeldt, V, Blievernicht, D, Bruce, R & Gilliam, T (1978). Joint Legislative Study on youth sport programs, Phase II: Agency-sponsored sports: Michigan state legislature, Lansing, MI.

Sisjord, MK (1993). Idrett og ungdomskultur (Sport and Youth culture). Norwegian University of Sport & Physical Education, Oslo. Doctoral thesis.

Skard, O. & Vaglum, P. (1989). The influence of psycosocial and sport factors on drop-out from boys' soccer. A prospective study. Scandinavian Journal of Sport Sciences 11, 65-72.

Smith, RE, Smoll, FL & Curtis, B (1979). Coach effectiveness training: A cognitive-behavioral approach to enhancing relationship skills in youth sport coaches. J of Sport Psychology, 1, 59-75.

Snyder, ML, Stephan, WG & Rosenfield, D (1978). Attributional egotism. In: Harvey, JH, Ickes, W and Kidd, RF (Eds.). New directions in attribution research vol. 2. pp. 91-120. Hillsdale NJ: Lawrence Erlbaum Associates.

Stipek, D & Mc Iver, D (1989). Developmental change in children's assessment of intelectual competence. Child Development, 60, 521-538.

Toda, M, Shinotsuka, H, Mc Clintock, CG & Stech, FJ (1978) Development of competitive behavior as a function of culture, age, and social comparison. J of Personality and Social Psychology, 36, 825-839.

Thill, E & Brunel, P (1995). Cognitive theories of motivation in sport. In: European Perspectives on exercise and sport psychology. Biddle,STH (Ed). Leeds, UK, Human Kinetics. (pp.195-217).

Treasure, DC & Roberts, GC (1995). Applications of achievement goal theory to physical education. Quest, 47, 475-489.

Veroff, J (1969). Social comparison and the development of acheivement motivation. In: Smith, CP (Ed.). Achievement related motives in children. pp. 46-101. New York: Russell Sage Foundation.

Walling, MD, Duda, JL & Chi, L (1993). The perceived motivational climate in sport questionnaire: Construct and predictive validity. J of Sport and Exercise Psychology, 15, 172-183.

Wankel, LM & Kreisel, PSJ (1985). Factors underlying enjoyment of youth sports: Sport and age group comparisons. Journal of Sport Psychology, 7, 51-64.

Wankel, LM & Sefton, JM (1989). A season-long investigation of fun in youth sports. J of Sport & Exercise Psychology, 11, 355-366.

Weiss, MR (1987). Self-esteem and achievement in children's sport and physical activity. In: Gould, D & Weiss, MR (Eds.). Advances in sport pediatrics, vol. 2, behavioral issues. pp. 87-119. Champaign, Illinois: Human Kinetics.

Weiss, M (1993). Psychlogical effects of intensive sport participation on children and youth: self-esteem and motivation. In: Intensive participation in children's sports, Cahill, BR & Pearl, AJ (Eds), Champaign: Illinois, Human Kinetics. pp. 39-70.

Weiss MR, Petlichkoff L (1989). Children's motivation for participation in and withdrawal from sport: Identifying the missing links. Pediatric Exercise Science, 1, 195-211.

Weiss, M, Ebbeck, V, McAuley, E, and Wiese, DM (1990). Self-esteem and causal attributions for children's physical and social competence in sport. J of Sport and Exercise Psychology, 12, 21-36.

Weiss, M & Chaumeton, N (1992). Motivational orientations in sport. In: Horn, TS (Ed). Advances in sport psychology. Champaign Illinois: Human Kinetics pp. 61-99.

Weitzer, JE (1989). Childhood socialization into physical activity: Parental roles in perceptions of competence and goal orientation. Unpublished masters thesis. University of Wisconsin at Milwaukee.

White, R. (1959). Motivation reconsidered: The concept of competence. Psychological Review, 66, 297-323.

Whitehead, J & Dalby, RA (1987). The development of effort and ability attributions in sport. Paper presented at a conference of the institute for the study of children in sport, Bedford College of Higher Education.

Wold, B (1989). Lifestyles and physical activity. A theoretical and empirical analysis of socialization among children and adolescents. Doctoral Thesis. Bergen: Department of psychology, University of Bergen.